Overdiagnosis of thyroid cancer in Fukushima

Sanae Midorikawa

Toru Takano

Akira Ohtsuru

Vicki J Schnadig

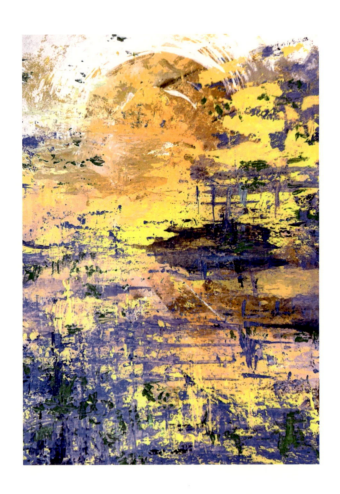

Sincere thanks to everyone who has cooperated with us to resolve the thyroid examination problem in Fukushima

Cover: **Hisui**

Authors

Sanae Midorikawa, M.D., PhD.

Professor (Clinical Medicine),
Miyagi Gakuin Women's University, Japan

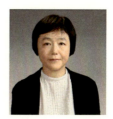

Dr. Midorikawa graduated from Fukushima Medical University in 1993. She has worked as a clinical endocrinologist for more than 20 years at Fukushima Medical University Hospital and related hospitals. After the Fukushima nuclear accident, she was involved in the thyroid cancer screening as a health surveillance for several years. She faced various issues related to thyroid cancer overdiagnosis. She has been engaged in communicating with residents and educating medical and non-medical students regarding thyroid cancer overdiagnosis. She reported the growth pattern of thyroid cancer diagnosed from thyroid cancer screening in children and young adults. She has been a core member of the Japan Consortium of Juvenile Thyroid Cancer (JCJTC) and a co-representative of NPO, POFF (Preventing Overdiagnosis from Fukushima) since 2020.

Toru Takano, M.D., PhD.

Director,
Thyroid Center, Rinku General Medical Center;
Guest Associate Professor,
Osaka University Graduate School of Medicine, Japan

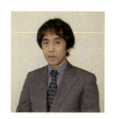

Dr. Takano first reported the gene expression profile of thyroid cancer and proposed a new theory of thyroid carcinogenesis, the fetal cell carcinogenesis theory, in 2000. The model he proposed for the natural history of thyroid cancer is now widely known. He was a member of the Prefectural Oversight Committee for the Fukushima Health Management Survey and the Task Force for Thyroid Examination from 2017 to 2019. He was a member of the Task Force for the European Thyroid Association Management Guidelines for Children with Thyroid Nodules and Differentiated Thyroid Cancer from 2019 to 2022. He has been a core member of the JCJTC since 2020.

Akira Ohtsuru, M.D., PhD.

Visiting Professor,
Atomic Bomb Disease Institute, Nagasaki University, Japan

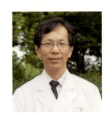

Dr. Ohtsuru graduated from Nagasaki University School of Medicine in 1982. He has worked as an internist in the 1st Department of Internal Medicine, Nagasaki University Hospital and related hospitals. He has researched the molecular mechanism of radiation-related carcinogenesis at the Atomic Bomb Disease Institute, Nagasaki University. He has worked as an associate professor of internal medicine at Nagasaki University Hospital to provide medical care for Hibakusha. He has been the professor of Department of Radiation Health Management, Fukushima Medical University since 2011 and the director of Radiation Disaster Medical Center, Fukushima University Hospital. He has worked as one of a core members in implementing the Fukushima Health Management Survey including the thyroid examination. He has been a core member of the JCJTC and a co-representative of POFF since 2020.

Vicki J Schnadig, M.D.

Professor Emerita (Pathology),
University of Texas Medical Branch, U.S.A.

Dr. Schnadig graduated from Northwestern University Medical School in 1975. She is American Board of Pathology certified in Anatomic and Clinical Pathology and has Special Competency/Added Qualification Board certification in Medical Microbiology and Cytopathology. Her major field of specialization is cytopathology. She has witnessed the explosion of fine-needle aspirations and surgeries performed for image-detected thyroid nodules in the United States and has become concerned about the physical, psychosocial and financial problems associated with overdiagnosis, overtreatment, and overuse of imaging. In 2020, she became an international advisory member of the JCJTC.

Contents*

Preface *1*

Endorsement *4*

Abbreviations *5*

Chapter 1
Overview of thyroid cancer overdiagnosis in children and adolescents *7*
Section 1
The mechanism that causes overdiagnosis in thyroid cancer: Self-limiting cancer as the cause of overdiagnosis *8*
Section 2
The use of thyroid US in asymptomatic children and adolescents *11*
Section 3
The harms of thyroid cancer overdiagnosis in the young *13*
Section 4
How the popularity paradox promotes false belief in the benefits of screening *14*
Section 5
Screening as a national project promotes overdiagnosis *15*
Column
Before performing thyroid FNAC on children, the risk-benefit ratio must be considered! *19*

Chapter 2
Overview of the thyroid examination in Fukushima *22*
Section 1
How was the thyroid examination started? *23*
Section 2
How the thyroid examination is carried out?
   1. Participation in the thyroid examination *26*
   2. School examination *27*
   3. Do subjects undergo the examination because they think it is necessary? *28*
   4. Problems with how to explain the results *29*
   5. The subjects of the thyroid examination were not informed of the purpose,

benefits or potential harms (risks) of the study *30*
Section 3
Summary of the results of the thyroid examination during 2011-2023 *32*

Chapter 3
What happened to the children after taking the thyroid examination? *36*
Section 1
Confusion caused by the category "A2" *37*
Section 2
What happened to the children who were diagnosed to have a thyroid nodule? *38*
Section 3
Impact of publicizing the examination results *39*
Section 4
Impact of results on examinees' sense of security and misunderstanding *40*
Section 5
What happened when the thyroid examination found cancer? *41*

Chapter 4
Overdiagnosis of thyroid cancer in Fukushima: How did it start and expand? *45*
Section 1
The origins of a huge thyroid cancer screening program *46*
Section 2
The FHMS leadership had high hopes, but the results were not what they expected *47*
Section 3
Controversy regarding thyroid cancer, is it radiation-induced or caused by screening effect? *48*
Section 4
The results of the second round confirmed the outbreak of overdiagnosis *48*
Section 5
Prediction of the number of cases detected in the FHMS in the future *51*
Section 6
Discussion by experts on thyroid cancer overdiagnosis in Fukushima Prefecture *51*
Section 7
The damages of overdiagnosis are now spreading outside the FHMS *56*

Chapter 5
Disagreements among academicians regarding the thyroid ultrasound examination and overdiagnosis *61*
Section 1
Recommendations by international organizations *62*
Section 2
The Japanese academic societies' viewpoints *64*
Section 3
Statement from the Science Council of Japan *65*
Section 4
Biased tone in Japanese academic journals *65*
Section 5
Conflicts in Japanese thyroid-related academic societies *67*
Section 6
Establishment of the Japan Consortium of Juvenile Thyroid Cancer *69*
Section 7
Reports from international organizations *70*
Section 8
Discussions on the IARC's recommendations *72*
Section 9
Discussions on active surveillance and the use of the term "overdiagnosis" *73*

Chapter 6
Contributions of politicians, political activists and the general public to the Fukushima overdiagnosis and overtreatment controversy *78*
Section 1
Residents and citizen groups *79*
Section 2
The politicians weigh in *81*
Section 3
Media and publishers *82*

Chapter 7
Personal perspectives of physicians directly involved in the Fukushima thyroid ultrasound examination *87*

Section 1
Start of the thyroid examination from the perspective of a medical doctor in Fukushima
  1. Situation before the thyroid examination and implementation of a new screening program (2011) *88*
  2. How the thyroid US examination was initiated (2011-2013) *89*
  3. Thyroid cancers were found in the confirmatory examination (2012-2014) *92*
  4. Efforts to lessen thyroid examination-related anxiety (2015) *94*
  5. Thoughts of an expert who led the thyroid examination: Dr. Shigenobu Nagataki *94*

Section 2
Confronting the problem of overdiagnosis and subsequent efforts to resolve it
  1. Overdiagnosis was first pointed out in Fukushima (2014) *97*
  2. Struggle to reduce the harm of overdiagnosis (2015-2021)
     1) Midorikawa and Ohtsuru's view on the overdiagnosis of thyroid cancer during the years 2015-2017 *99*
     2) Challenges to solve the problem of overdiagnosis (2015) *102*
     3) Attempt to modify the test methods to prevent overdiagnosis (2015-2017) *103*
     4) Forces against efforts to curb overdiagnosis (2017-2021) *106*

Section 3
What does the thyroid examination mean to each person involved?
  1. Children do not want their caregivers to be sad *109*
  2. Emotional conflict among medical staff involved in the thyroid examination *110*
  3. Problems with media coverage in Fukushima *113*
  4. Difficulty in modifying the thyroid examination by personnel affiliated with FMU *115*

Chapter 8
How to educate about cancer overdiagnosis? *122*
Section 1
Teaching about overdiagnosis in medical and allied health schools
  1. Need for education of physicians and medical students *124*
  2. Materials for the education of medical students *125*

Section 2
How does one implement educational change in academic societies? *126*

Section 3
How to and what to discuss with the public, residents, and patients to make them understand overdiagnosis: From the experience in Fukushima

1. People tend to overestimate the benefits of screening and medical intervention *128*
2. Use of explanatory meetings for parents and other residents with the intent to reduce anxiety *129*
3. Use of classroom dialogues with children *130*
4. Need for personal interaction with subjects *131*
5. Necessity of debating harms and benefits *131*
6. Use of social media to educate the public *132*
7. What should we discuss with patients? *133*
8. Patients' and clinicians' discomfort with overdiagnosis discussion *134*
9. Complicated situation in Fukushima *134*
10. Summary *135*

Chapter 9
Summary of discussion points and proposals for the future *140*
Section 1
What should we reflect on? *141*
Section 2
Measures to mitigate the harms of screening-induced overdiagnosis *144*

Afterword *150*

*The views expressed in this book are those of the authors and do not represent the views of any institutions to which they are affiliated.

Preface

This book is based on the book published by Akebishobo in 2021 entitled "Thyroid examination in Fukushima and overdiagnosis: What can we do for the children?" The original book was in Japanese and for the general public. We extracted information for experts, rewrote it, and translated it into English.

Thyroid cancer screening started in Japan after the Fukushima Daiichi Nuclear Power Plant accident in 2011. The related overdiagnosis has afflicted more than 300 children and adolescents, and the damage continues to grow. The reason is apparent. Until 2024, the thyroid screening program in Fukushima is still executing without any changes from its start despite the damage. Overseas experts may wonder why it goes like this.

Since ancient times, the most cherished concept in Japanese society was "conformity." The Japanese word representing conformity is "wa," not surprisingly, which is the same word meaning "Japan." Japanese people tend to flow in one direction as a group. It is a great advantage when trying to reach one big goal together. However, when a national prestige project turns out to be wrong, it becomes hard to turn around. In other countries, many discussions may be exchanged, and improvements may be sought in such a case. In Japan, on the contrary, much effort is made to justify the outcome and seal the arguments that can be the source of conflict, saying, "Don't try to find faults with others!"

It's undoubtedly embarrassing, but for this reason, Japan is said to be an overdiagnosis powerhouse. When Japan suffered from overdiagnosis of infant neuroblastoma, the screening continued for over thirty years. It was not until the domestic experts were exposed to bitter criticism from overseas that the harm of its overdiagnosis finally ceased. Overdiagnosis of thyroid cancer in Fukushima is likely to follow a similar path. Therefore, it is our urgent task to confer the present situation in Japan with overseas experts.

Now we recognize that thyroid cancer overdiagnosis in children was first experienced in the countries around Chornobyl. As described in this book, Japan has significantly contributed to implementing the thyroid ultrasound screening at Chornobyl. However, the information on overdiagnosis was blocked locally due to the movement to justify such medical practice. That such experience was not shared internationally led to the spread of damage in Fukushima.

This book describes in detail the behavior of those involved in the thyroid examination in Fukushima. We want to emphasize that it is not written to accuse anyone. The purpose is to leave a detailed record of the incident and use it to evaluate what was right and wrong later. Furthermore, what is happening in Fukushima is the overdiagnosis of cancer caused by a school check-up, which is the first experience in history. This experience should be recorded in detail and passed on to posterity so that it will never be repeated. We have avoided mentioning the names of those whose actions have become a factor in exacerbating the problem. Instead, we have listed the literature so the reader can investigate the situation.

Moreover, this incident is critical as teaching material for studying medical ethics. Suppose medical students learn about particular happenings in the Fukushima thyroid cancer overdiagnosis. In that case, they will sympathize with some related people and dislike others. Also, they will think about what they would do if they were in a position actually to be in charge of the examination at the site. Such thought experiments give students a valuable opportunity to think about how they should be as medical professionals.

Allow me to write about my personal experience on this issue. I was the one who first wrote a paper that thyroid cancer is already formed in childhood. I might be the only one, as a Japanese researcher, who really benefited from the start of the thyroid examination in Fukushima because, as a result, my research work became known worldwide. Although I foresaw the outcome quite precisely, at first, I stood by and just watched the growing damage in Fukushima because I was optimistic that the leading researchers in Japan would change their minds after seeing the data obtained and work spontaneously to solve the problem. But the actual situation was not so. Even after I became directly involved in the thyroid examination as one of the members of the expert board of Fukushima Prefecture, I could not change the minds of other experts who insisted that the thyroid examination benefits children. When I think about the still ongoing project in Fukushima, instead of feeling happy that my research has been acknowledged, I feel guilty for not being able to stop it. For me, writing this book meant redemption.

From this viewpoint, I greatly respect the two authors, Sanae Midorikawa and Akira Ohtsuru. They were the chief members that carried out the thyroid examination in Fukushima. However, they realized early on the harm of overdiagnosis and did not hesitate to warn the residents. Unfortunately, as described in this book, they had to quit their jobs. When we planned this book, they hesitated to write about Fukushima's events in detail since such work might remind them of what they had faced, which was very painful. However, documenting their experience was necessary to assess Fukushima's events. So even though I realized it was challenging for them, I finally persuaded them to agree to write it. In this book, they provided truthful information on what was going on at the thyroid examination site. Without their courageous decision, the value of this book would have been greatly reduced.

In this book, Chapters 2, 3, 7 and a part of 8 were mainly written by Drs. Midorikawa and Ohtsuru, and I was the principal author of Chapters 1, 4-6, 9 and a part of 8. Dr. Schnadig was responsible for overall supervision. She has reworked many parts of the text in this book. We, the Japanese authors, needed to have English proofreading by experts who understood the complex and multifaceted problem of overdiagnosis. Without hesitation, we asked Dr. Schnadig to take on this role because she had written a paper that expressed an accurate opinion on overdiagnosis, and the English text of the article was incredibly moving for us. She has always been a constant ally in our fight against overdiagnosis and encouraged us a lot when we put this book together. Her advice has always been a source of inspiration to us.

Finally, the authors thank Shinichi Okabayashi, President of Akebishobo, the publisher. He is the one who planned to publish the Japanese book on thyroid cancer overdiagnosis in Fukushima four years ago when other publishers were not yet interested in this issue. We could start this project because of this solid support.

Be aware that this book was completed with the courage and goodwill of many. All the authors hope that the information in this book will help prevent the spread of damage caused by thyroid cancer overdiagnosis, not only in Japan but worldwide. Please remind that Fukushima's damage continues to expand even today, and urgent countermeasures are needed.

Toru Takano
Rinku General Medical Center,
Japan

Endorsement

I highly commend this thoughtful account of the Fukushima Health Management Survey thyroid cancer screening program, started after the Fukushima Daiichi Nuclear Power Plant accident in 2011. Although motivated by good intentions, emerging evidence showed that the program was harming rather than benefiting children. Along with the harms of thyroid cancer overdiagnosis, the authors identify multiple ethical issues including lack of fully informed consent, normalization of screening, conflicts of interest, special interest campaigns, and both political and professional unwillingness to revise the screening program in the light of new evidence. The authors provide fascinating insights into how these ethical issues unfolded and the challenges of countering mistaken beliefs and ingrained assumptions about the benefits of early diagnosis. The book is an excellent and detailed case study on potential ethical pitfalls of screening. In addition, it provides practical and ethically robust suggestions for reducing current and ongoing harms of the program.

Wendy Rogers BM.BS, BAHons, PhD, MRCGP, FRACGP, FAHA
Distinguished Professor, Department of Philosophy and School of Medicine, Macquarie University;
Co-Director, Macquarie University Ethics and Agency Research Centre, Australia

Abbreviations

AS active surveillance
CT computed tomography
EU European Union
FHMS Fukushima Health Management Survey[1]

[1]Soon after the earthquake and nuclear accident on March 2011, Fukushima Prefecture launched the FHMS to investigate radiation exposure level caused by the accident and direct/indirect health effects. Fukushima Medical University took the lead in planning and implementing this survey.

FMU Fukushima Medical University[2]

[2]FMU was founded on 1944 for the purpose of nurturing medical professionals in Fukushima Prefecture. After that, a graduate school, university hospitals, affiliated research institutes, and the faculties of nursing and health sciences were gradually established in addition to the medical school. FMU is an only medical university in Fukushima Prefecture.

FNAC fine-needle aspiration cytology
IARC International Agency for Research on Cancer
JCJTC Japan Consortium of Juvenile Thyroid Cancer
JTA Japan Thyroid Association
MeSH Medical Subjects Headings
NTI needle tract implantation
PMC papillary microcarcinoma
POCF Prefectural Oversight Committee for the FHMS[3]

[3]This committee was established by Fukushima Prefecture to provide oversight advice from a professional standpoint on the FHMS.

POFF Preventing Overdiagnosis from Fukushima
PTC papillary thyroid carcinoma
SCJ Science Council of Japan
SCO Save Children from Overdiagnosis
SLC self-limiting cancer
SHAMISEN
Nuclear Emergency Situation-Improvement of Medical and Health Surveillance
TBS Tokyo Broadcasting System Television
TEPCO Tokyo Electric Power Company Holdings
TFTE Task Force for Thyroid Examination[4]

[4]This committee was established by Fukushima Prefecture to analyze and discuss the data of the thyroid examination.

TM-NUC Thyroid Health Monitoring after Nuclear Accidents
TUE thyroid ultrasound examination
US ultrasound
USPSTF United States Preventive Service Task Force
WHO World Health Organization

Chapter 1
Overview of thyroid cancer overdiagnosis in children and adolescents

In order to fully comprehend the material presented in this book, it is important to understand the current meaning of the term "overdiagnosis". For many years, overdiagnosis meant a misdiagnosis or diagnostic error. Aronson has written an excellent review of the history and current usage of the term.[1] Recently, overdiagnosis has been redefined. The National Library of Medicine has included overdiagnosis in its Medical Subjects Headings (MeSH). Overdiagnosis means "labeling of a person with a disease or abnormal condition that would not have caused the person harm if left undiscovered." The MeSH definition includes expanding the prevalence of disease by lowering the threshold for diagnosis or widening diagnostic criteria without proof that these expansions actually help the patient.[2] In addition to defining overdiagnosis, the MeSH entry offers a warning that patients not only receive no benefit from overdiagnosis but may "experience physical, psychological, or financial harm."

In 2010, Welch and Black introduced readers to overdiagnosis in cancer, meaning "diagnosis of a [cancer] that would otherwise not go on to cause symptoms or death."[3] These authors emphasized that there are two overdiagnosis prerequisites: the existence of a subclinical reservoir of these "cancers" and activities (such as screening by imaging or blood testing) that lead to cancer detection. However, the concept of overdiagnosis of cancer remains difficult for the general public to understand. Thyroid cancer is very prone to overdiagnosis because of the increased use of sensitive radiologic imaging and the presence of a sizable pool of indolent, subclinical thyroid tumors.

This chapter explains how thyroid cancer overdiagnosis occurs and summarizes the various phenomena associated with thyroid cancer overdiagnosis in children and adolescents. The chapter also discusses the most recent theory concerning the mechanism of thyroid cancer initiation and progression, which is quite different from previously published theories. This new information includes the concept of indolent or non-progressive cancers (self-limiting cancers, SLCs) and explains the susceptibility of thyroid cancer to overdiagnosis. In the 21st century, there is a need to redefine cancer. There is conclusive evidence that not all cancers are the aggressive, inevitably fatal diseases they were once believed to be.

Section 1
The mechanism that causes overdiagnosis in thyroid cancer: Self-limiting cancer as the cause of overdiagnosis

Recent studies have revealed a more complete understanding of the natural history of thyroid cancer. These studies have overturned the conventional concept of cancer.[4] In South Korea, widespread implementation of ultrasound (US) thyroid screening found many small thyroid cancers. As a result, the diagnosis of thyroid cancer increased 15-fold. Most patients underwent surgery; however, thyroid cancer-related mortality did not decrease thereafter.[5] This finding provides evidence that small thyroid cancers found by US screening do not cause cancer-related deaths.

Data from observational trials of papillary microcarcinoma (PMC) support this conclusion. Globally, active surveillance (AS) is becoming an acceptable alternative to immediate surgery for PMC of 1cm or less. Ito *et al.* found very low rates of tumor progression in PMC followed by AS.[6] Most progression occurred in patients younger than 40 years, and no deaths or transformation to anaplastic carcinoma were observed. Thousands of patients have already undergone such follow-up, but no one has died from cancer, and no PMC has been reported to transform into more malignant forms such as anaplastic carcinoma.

Given that most papillary thyroid carcinomas (PTCs) grow very slowly, even in young adults, initiation of these tumors is likely to occur in infancy. It is hypothesized that PTCs develop in infancy or early childhood and undergo a transient period of rapid growth usually followed by slowing growth or complete proliferation arrest. Such an assumption was supported by examining thyroid cancers found by US in children in Fukushima. It is known that during the teenage years, the incidence of small thyroid cancer rapidly increases with age. Midorikawa *et al.* found that during the observation period, thyroid carcinomas did not grow or increase in volume in a linear fashion and fell into a growth arrest phase after an initial period of cell proliferation.[7] Their findings suggest that US screening may be detecting many subclinical PTCs not destined to progress to clinical significance. It is also important to note that pathologic examination of resected childhood PMC with node dissection has often revealed local invasion or lymph node metastases.[8] What still remains unknown, given the overall excellent prognosis of childhood PTC, is the clinical significance of subclinical lymph node or even distant metastases.

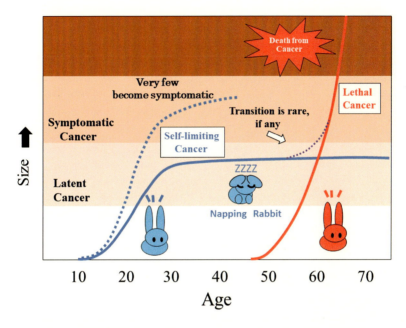

Fig. 1-1 Natural history of thyroid cancer based on the recent evidence

Thyroid cancer in children and adolescents is often found in an advanced state. For example, children often present with large nodules and lymph node or lung metastases. However, despite the presence of local or distant metastasis, the prognosis is excellent, and patients rarely die of thyroid cancer.[9] Juvenile thyroid cancer is like the rabbit in the Aesop fable. When the rabbit competed in a race with the turtle, it began to run at a fierce speed but eventually got tired, took a nap, and consequently lost to the turtle. Similarly, juvenile thyroid cancer proliferates actively and spreads locally or, in some cases, distantly in its early stages of development. However, its growth slows down, and then it takes a nap (Fig. 1-1). Some researchers call this "napping rabbit" self-limiting cancer (SLC).[10] It is pathologically "cancer" because it metastasizes; however, it should be treated more like a benign tumor as it rarely kills the patient. The existence of SLC is challenging to understand because the classical multistep carcinogenesis theory tells us that if a tumor is left untreated, it becomes more aggressive due to the accumulation of new genetic alternations.[11] Both physicians and the lay population have traditionally been taught that cancer screening, early diagnosis and treatment are beneficial, and it is difficult to change these beliefs.

Some researchers claim that thyroid cancers which lead to cancer-related death are derived from PMCs.[12] According to the data from Japanese health check-ups, 0.5% of adults have small thyroid cancers that can only be found by US, and in Japan, 0.1% of deaths are due to thyroid cancer.[13] If the above hypothesis is correct, one out of five people with a small thyroid cancer will die of thyroid cancer. This calculation does not explain why surgical removal of small thyroid cancers did not decrease thyroid cancer-related mortality in South Korea.[5] Furthermore, although thousands of patients with a PMC have undergone AS, none of them died of thyroid cancer.[6] Thus, it should be concluded that SLC rarely, if ever, turns into more aggressive cancer.

About 10% of patients with thyroid cancer die of thyroid cancer. This indicates that there exists another type of thyroid cancer that is different from SLC.[4] This cancer is called lethal thyroid cancer.[10] Its nature can be predicted from epidemiological data. Since the prognosis of juvenile thyroid cancer is excellent, lethal cancer occurs almost entirely in the elderly. Given the experience from South Korea and AS, lethal cancer is rarely found as a small nodule because of its early aggressive growth pattern. Therefore, it is usually found as a large nodule accompanied by clinical symptoms. Unlike SLC, lethal cancer grows unremittingly, leading to cancer-related death.[10]

Lethal cancer and SLC probably have different origins. Recent molecular analyses support this conclusion. Some believe that anaplastic carcinoma arises via genetic mutations in indolent, differentiated carcinomas.[11] However, comprehensive analyses of genetic alterations in anaplastic carcinoma accompanying differentiated carcinoma reveal that many genetic abnormalities found in differentiated carcinoma are not found in the co-existing anaplastic carcinoma. This indicates that, although these two cancers may co-exist, they develop independently.[14-16] The idea that differentiated carcinoma cells evolve into anaplastic carcinoma cells may not be correct. More likely, anaplastic carcinomas arise from persisting primitive, stem cell-like remnants within differentiated tumors. These primitive cells (or fetal cells), which are different from the cells found in SLC, suddenly begin unregulated proliferation in elderly patients (Fig. 1-2).[17]

Based on what is now known about the differences in clinical behavior, genetic composition, and age of onset of differentiated and anaplastic thyroid carcinomas, it can be concluded that thyroid cancer overdiagnosis has become such a serious problem because most PTCs are SLC. In the classical multistep carcinogenesis theory, there is considerable risk for the acquisition of new mutations leading to aggressive behavior or death if cancers are left untreated. The concept of SLC is difficult for both patients and physicians to accept because, traditionally, both have been taught that early diagnosis and treatment are always justified. Many clinicians still adhere to the classical multistep carcinogenesis theory and refuse to accept the concept of overdiagnosis.

It is difficult to reconcile the natural history of thyroid cancer with the classical multistep carcinogenesis theory. As described above, tumors from different origins show unique growth patterns in the thyroid, and there is no evident benign to malignant progression. These phenomena can be better explained by the fetal cell carcinogenesis theory, which states that thyroid tumors develop directly from the remnants of various fetal thyroid cells formed during the time of thyroid development.[18]

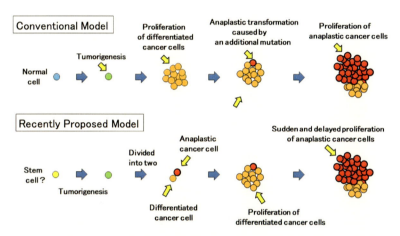

Fig. 1-2 Conventional and recently proposed models of anaplastic transformation

Section 2
The use of thyroid US in asymptomatic children and adolescents

Considering the natural history of thyroid cancer mentioned in the previous section, the rationale for- and consequences of using thyroid US in asymptomatic children and adolescents are summarized as follows: It is generally believed that early diagnosis can prevent cancer death and reduce the rate of recurrence. However, such desirable effects have not been confirmed in thyroid US screening of asymptomatic children and adolescents. The prognosis of thyroid cancer in children is excellent, with a 30-year survival rate of 99%.[19] Early diagnosis cannot improve the prognosis.

Hay et al. wrote an important paper dealing with whether early diagnosis by thyroid US reduces the recurrence rate of PTC. These authors analyzed the clinical data of thyroid cancers in children without metastasis at the initial surgery and compared the recurrence rates before and after the introduction of US. Before the introduction of US, there was almost no recurrence, but after the introduction, recurrence was observed in over 10 and 50% of the cases 10 and 30 years after surgery, respectively.[19]

The cause of this striking difference is not clear yet. However, there are some theoretical reasons. First, overdiagnosis of recurrence should be considered. The use of US and other sensitive imaging techniques followed by fine-needle aspiration cytology (FNAC) and surgery may identify clinically insignificant recurrences that were never found prior to the use of US and computed tomography (CT). In Fukushima's thyroid screening program, several patients had distant metastases. Although the number of patients with distant metastases was small, the rate per population is about 50-fold higher than reported in the United States.[20] In other words, Fukushima US thyroid screening and use of follow-up radiologic imaging, FNAC and surgery may be finding tumors with distant metastases that would never prove life-threatening or cause morbidity. Second, in order to preserve thyroid function and avoid criticism of overtreatment, simple hemithyroidectomy is often performed for the treatment of small PTC. Given that PTC often spreads non-lethally in young people, continued monitoring with US may later find clinically insignificant recurrences in the remaining thyroid gland.

Thyroid FNAC under US guidance has now become routine, and screening of children for thyroid nodules increases the number of children being referred for diagnostic FNAC. Although risk of serious complications caused by thyroid FNAC is low, this procedure can be frightening and traumatic for young children. The indications for FNAC of small, suspicious thyroid nodules in children should be considered more carefully so as to minimize unneeded procedures, and FNAC should not be performed unless surgery is planned based on the results. Our concerns regarding FNAC will be discussed in the column at the end of this chapter.

Thus, the idea that early diagnosis and treatment of thyroid cancer in the young leads to improved quality of life (QOL) is too optimistic. One should remember that most PTCs are SLC. Surgery during the asymptomatic stage is mostly overtreatment or surgery performed too early. In the latter case, a recurrence found after thyroidectomy leading to a second surgical procedure. In both instances, the surgical procedures may be unnecessary if the tumor and recurrences are subclinical. Therefore, few patients benefit from surgery. As described in the next section, the harm of overdiagnosis of thyroid cancer is far more severe in children and adolescents than in adults.

Overall, early diagnosis of thyroid cancer by US has no apparent benefit, while it causes harm from overdiagnosis or surgery too early; thus, the harms outweigh the benefits.

Section 3
The harms of thyroid cancer overdiagnosis in the young[21]

Patients often elect to undergo cancer screening even when informed about the risks of false positives and detection of subclinical, indolent "cancers" that will not progress during their lifetimes (overdiagnosis). Also, patients may choose surgery rather than AS because, both to them and their physicians, the word "cancer" means a lethal condition requiring excision. Pressure to undergo surgery from family and physicians may make opting for AS very difficult.[22] The potential for unnecessary surgery is even higher for children whose dutiful parents cannot allow their children to go untreated after a cancer diagnosis. In fact, most children diagnosed with thyroid cancer in Fukushima have already had surgery.[8] Thus, children undergo unnecessary surgery with the risk of surgical complications or need for lifetime thyroid hormone replacement.

AS, long-term observation without surgery, can be especially burdensome for children. It is known that thyroid cancer in the young can recur several decades after surgery; therefore, AS should be continued virtually for life.[19] We do not have evidence that asymptomatic PTC with lymph node or distant metastases reduces survival. Yet, the concept of indolent or harmless metastasis contradicts all that patients and physicians have been taught and is not yet widely accepted. During AS, the detection of a small increase in the nodule size or a small metastasis can generate new worries and the need for decisions regarding whether to have surgery. Because it is not yet generally accepted that AS of asymptomatic metastatic cancers is a safe option, AS of children may be regarded as a form of child abuse or neglect. It should be noted that the harm of overdiagnosis begins with the *diagnosis* of cancer, and it continues whether or not patients undergo surgery.

Overdiagnosis of thyroid cancer in children and adolescents is more of a human rights problem than a health problem.[23, 24] The general public regard childhood cancer as a lethal disease. Regardless of the excellent prognosis of juvenile thyroid cancer, children and adolescents may suffer from discrimination and stigmatization after diagnosis. They will be trying to finish school, get a job, get married, and have children after being labeled as cancer patients. When thyroid cancer is found after a nuclear accident, there is potential for the mistaken belief that radiation exposure puts them at high risk for developing cancer. The families of the children diagnosed with thyroid cancer in Fukushima are more concerned about whether their children will be able to marry than their health problems.[23] They also suffer financial disadvantages. In many cases, they are refused insurance or loans. These situations cause significant stress for children.

Although childhood thyroid cancer is not usually life-threatening, the QOL of children diagnosed with thyroid cancer declines, and the negative impact on educational performance is particularly significant.[25] In summary, thyroid cancer *diagnosis* can be more threatening to children than thyroid cancer itself.

Section 4
How the popularity paradox promotes false belief in the benefits of screening

Raffle and Grey noted an ironic consequence of cancer screening programs, which they called "the popularity paradox."[26] The popularity paradox occurs in screening programs where there is a high rate of overdiagnosis and subsequent overtreatment. Patients who screen positive for a condition and are treated for that condition believe that their lives were saved by screening and intervention. They do not recognize that their excellent outcomes were due to the detection of harmless lesions (that they were overdiagnosed). Hence, the higher the rate of overdiagnosis, the more people believe in the health benefits of screening and promote screening to others. In general, patients are more afraid of missed diagnoses than overdiagnosis, and physicians fear patient anger and litigation. This leads to excessive use of highly sensitive screening tools and to more overdiagnosis and false positives.

Around the globe, physicians and other healthcare workers are beginning to recognize the need to orchestrate programs to explain the concept of overdiagnosis to patients in language that they can understand and to deal with patient confusion or anger. People generally believe that an early cancer diagnosis always does them good. It is difficult for physicians who have made a diagnosis to tell their patients that the diagnosis is meaningless. Surgeons are unlikely to tell patients that they removed a cancer unnecessarily. Benefits and risks and the concept of indolent "cancers" must be discussed prior to screening and treatment. Patients who are status post-cancer diagnosis and treatment are not likely to be receptive to being told that they have been "overdiagnosed." Even when informed of the concept of overdiagnosis and desirous of AS, patients' families and physicians may pressure patients to have surgery.[22]

We are seeing the popularity paradox in Fukushima. There have been no requests to stop the thyroid US examination among patients diagnosed with thyroid cancer. Some citizens' groups emphasize that patients recommend continuing the thyroid US examination because it enables them to find their cancers early.

Section 5
Screening as a national project promotes overdiagnosis

Large health surveys that include screening of a mixed population of subjects often detect subclinical, harmless conditions, thus triggering overdiagnosis and overtreatment. A large budget is allocated to these surveys that are led by authoritative experts. Once money, professional reputations, and news coverage have been devoted to these projects, it is difficult to admit mistakes and stop or modify the programs even when data emerges that the projects are more harmful than beneficial. Misleading, one-sided information that is not justified by the science may be disseminated via news or social media, promoting the survey's benefits and failing to adequately explain its harms. Conflicting views on the project confuse the public, and failure to engage in productive discussions of benefits and harms allows for continuance of the project.

The following are some examples: In Japan, newborn mass screening for neuroblastoma was started in 1973. However, this test did not reduce the mortality of neuroblastoma. Discussions in Japanese academic societies did not progress quickly. It was not until overseas researchers published papers on the problem of overdiagnosis that the Japanese government started a discussion about whether or not to continue the examination. The examination ended after the people who started the project left the scene, at which point 30 years had passed. By this time, screening was being performed throughout Japan.[27]

When overdiagnosis following excessive use of thyroid US became a problem in South Korea after 2010, thyroid specialists denied the harm of thyroid US screening and insisted on continuing the examination. They argued that people should not be deprived of the opportunity for early diagnosis.[23, 28]

There is no doubt that the overdiagnosis of childhood thyroid cancer by US occurred following the Chornobyl disaster. After the nuclear plant accident, many

Japanese experts were dispatched to the areas contaminated with radioactive materials with funding from a Japanese foundation and helped with thyroid screening and surgery.[29] They are now praised and admired as Chornobyl's heroes for saving many children's lives.

The events that occurred in Chornobyl in 1986 are quite different from those in Fukushima in 2011. Radiation released at Chornobyl was much higher than at Fukushima, and in Chornobyl, there were fatalities owing to acute radiation syndrome.[29,30] Although it is agreed that the Chornobyl nuclear accident resulted in an increase in childhood PTC, there is a lack of evidence that radiation-induced PTC increases the risk of PTC death. Both radiation-induced and spontaneous PTC appear to be largely SLC. Thus, US screening in Chornobyl undoubtedly resulted in the detection of indolent, subclinical tumors and overdiagnosis. The indolence of these tumors is indicated by the 10-year survival rate of >99%.[30]

A study reported that, although the influence of the poor social environment cannot be excluded, children diagnosed with thyroid cancer after the Chornobyl accident were at a high risk of attempting suicide.[31] One wonders about the degree to which these cancer diagnoses contributed to stress and increased risks of suicide.

There has been little discussion of overdiagnosis in Chornobyl, and there have been, thus far, few publications concerning overdiagnosis in Chornobyl. PubMed search found eight documents using Chornobyl and overdiagnosis as keywords. The Chornobyl experience has not been put to good use in Fukushima, where US thyroid screening continues.

The history of medicine is filled with mistakes made by great physicians and researchers trying to help humankind. We must face the fact that harm can be caused by screening projects initiated with the best intentions. The leadership in these projects must humbly and openly acknowledge their mistakes and failures. Scientific, evidence-based data comparing benefits and harms must be calmly and openly discussed among experts. Most importantly, there should be no attempt to hide negative findings that do not support the project. The harms of overdiagnosis will continue to increase if leaders do not humbly admit mistakes, honestly inform the public of them, and take steps to stop or modify projects where the harms outweigh the benefits.[23, 24]

References

1. Aronson JK. When I use a word....too much healthcare-diagnosis. *BMJ* 378:o2062, 2022.

2. National Library of Medicine. U.S.A.: MeSH Overdiagnosis. [internet, cited 2024 July 15] Available from: https://www.ncbi.nlm.nih.gov/mesh/?term=overdiagnosis.
3. Welch HG, Black WC. Overdiagnosis in cancer. *J Natl Cancer Inst* 102:605-13, 2010.
4. Takano T. Natural history of thyroid cancer. *Endocr J* 64:237-44, 2017.
5. Ahn HS, et al. Korea's thyroid-cancer "epidemic"--screening and overdiagnosis. *N Engl J Med* 371:1765-7, 2014.
6. Ito Y, et al. Patient age is significantly related to the progression of papillary microcarcinoma of the thyroid under observation. *Thyroid* 24:27-34, 2014.
7. Midorikawa S, et al. Comparative analysis of the growth pattern of thyroid cancer in young patients screened by ultrasonography in Japan after a nuclear accident: The Fukushima Health Management Survey. *JAMA Otolaryngol Head Neck Surg* 144:57-63, 2018.
8. Suzuki S, et al. Histopathological analysis of papillary thyroid carcinoma detected during ultrasound screening examinations in Fukushima. *Cancer Sci* 110:817-27, 2019.
9. Rivkees SA, et al. The treatment of differentiated thyroid cancer in children: emphasis on surgical approach and radioactive iodine therapy. *Endocr Rev* 32:798-826, 2011.
10. Takano T. Overdiagnosis of juvenile thyroid cancer: Time to consider self-limiting cancer. *J Adolesc Young Adult Oncol* 9:286-8, 2020.
11. Kondo T, et al. Pathogenetic mechanisms in thyroid follicular-cell neoplasia. *Nat Rev Cancer* 24:292-306, 2006.
12. Williams D. Thyroid growth and cancer. *Eur Thyroid J* 4: 164-73, 2015.
13. Shimura H. Prevalence and clinical course of thyroid tumor in Japan: Data from medical checkups. *J Jpn Thyroid Assoc* 1:109-13 2010 (in Japanese).
14. Capdevila J, et al. Early evolutionary divergence between papillary and anaplastic thyroid cancers. *Ann Oncol* 29:1454-60, 2018.
15. Dong W, et al. Clonal evolution analysis of paired anaplastic and well-differentiated thyroid carcinomas reveals shared common ancestor. *Genes Chromosomes Cancer* 57:645-52, 2018.
16. Paulsson JO, et al. Whole-genome sequencing of synchronous thyroid carcinomas identifies aberrant DNA repair in thyroid cancer dedifferentiation. *J Pathol* 250:183–94, 2020.
17. Takano T. Fetal cell carcinogenesis of the thyroid: Theory and practice. *Semin Cancer Biol* 17:233-40, 2007.

18. Takano T. Fetal cell carcinogenesis of the thyroid: A modified theory based on recent evidence. *Endocr J* 61:311-20, 2014.
19. Hay ID, *et al*. Papillary thyroid carcinoma (PTC) in children and adults: Comparison of initial presentation and long-term postoperative outcome in 4432 patients consecutively treated at the Mayo Clinic during eight decades (1936–2015). *World J Surg* 42:329–42, 2018.
20. Takano T. Natural history of thyroid cancer suggests beginning of the overdiagnosis of juvenile thyroid cancer in the United State. *Cancer* 125: 4107-8, 2019.
21. Murakami M, *et al*. Harms of pediatric thyroid cancer overdiagnosis. *JAMA Otolaryngol Head Neck Surg* 146:84, 2020.
22. Davis L, *et al*. Experience of US patients who self-identify as having an overdiagnosed thyroid cancer: a qualitative analysis. *JAMA Otolaryngol Head Neck Surg* 143:663-9, 2017.
23. Takano T. Overdiagnosis of thyroid cancer in Fukushima. *J Society Risk Analysis, Japan* 28:67-76, 2019 (in Japanese).
24. Takano T. Overdiagnosis of juvenile thyroid cancer. *Eur Thyroid J* 9:124-31, 2020.
25. Perez MN, *et al*. Health-related quality of life at diagnosis for pediatric thyroid cancer patients. *J Clin Endocrinol Metab* 108:e169-e177, 2023.
26. Raffle AE, Gray JAM. Popularity paradox. In: Screening: evidence and practice. Oxford University Press, p.68, 2007.
27. Yamamichi T, *et al*. Result of mass screening for neuroblastoma in 18-month-old infants in Osaka area, Japan. *Pediatr Surg Int* 37:1645-9, 2021.
28. JoongAng Daily in Japanese. Korea: Thyroid cancer in Korean women is 14 times higher than in Japan. Why? (in Japanese) [internet, cited 2024 July 15] Available from: https://japanese.joins.com/JArticle/162430.
29. Nagataki S, Yamashita S. Thirty years after the Chernobyl Nuclear Power Plant Accident: Contribution from Japan—"Confirming the increase of childhood thyroid cancer." In: Thyroid cancer and nuclear accidents: Long-term aftereffects of Chernobyl and Fukushima (1st ed.). Academic Press, pp.11-20, 2017.
30. Thomas G, Yamashita S. Thirty years after Chernobyl and 5 after Fukushima-what have we learnt and what do we still need to know? In: Thyroid cancer and nuclear accidents: Long-term aftereffects of Chernobyl and Fukushima (1st ed.). Academic Press, xv-xxiv, 2017.
31. Fridman MV, *et al*. Clinical and morphological features of papillary thyroid cancer in children and adolescents in the Republic of Belarus: analysis of 936 post-Chernobyl carcinomas. *Vopr Onkol* 60:43-6, 2014 (in Russian).

[Column]
Before performing thyroid FNAC on children, the risk-benefit ratio must be considered!

FNAC has proven to be a very valuable, minimally invasive tool when used for diagnosis and triage of clinically evident masses or suspected metastases in patients with histories of aggressive neoplasms. FNAC allows for non-surgical management of non-neoplastic conditions as well as non-surgical treatment of some malignancies. There is no doubt that, when used selectively, FNAC can reduce unnecessary surgery and preclude the need for open biopsy. However, one must question the beneficence of FNAC when performed on subclinical, US-screen-detected thyroid nodules in children and adolescents. One must also question the beneficence of FNAC of subclinical, small metastases in childhood PTC. It is probable that most of these detected "cancers" are going to be self-limiting or indolent.[1,2]

Although there is a general consensus that risk for serious complications of thyroid FNAC is very low, there are deficits in the reporting of adverse effects. Publications reviewing thyroid FNAC tend to emphasize accuracy and value of the procedure and minimize, or fail to mention, complications. Also, there is variability in what are considered complications. Localized hematoma or ecchymosis formation, post-procedural pain and even vasovagal reactions have been considered minor or expected findings by some. Only conditions causing substantial morbidity, requiring additional therapy, hospitalization or prolonged hospitalization are consistently considered serious. These include severe bleeding, large, symptomatic hematoma, permanent nerve damage and needle tract implantation (NTI). Fortunately, all of these are exceedingly rare. There have been no prospective studies, to our knowledge, evaluating the psychological effects of FNAC on children or the reactions of care-takers to FNAC complications regarded as minor.

There have been few publications that focus directly on thyroid FNAC complications. Polyzos and Anastasilakis[3] performed a systematic review of complications of thyroid FNAC and concluded that although the overall safety of FNAC remains unquestioned, "physicians should always weigh the risk-benefit ratio on an individual basis before the procedure". These authors also mention that there is a lack of systematic reporting of post-FNAC complications. Heterogeneity of definitions, records, patient selection and publication bias, including non-acceptance of case reports, are likely contributing to underestimation of complications. Cappelli et al.[4] reported 10 complications out of 7449 needle aspirations and considered only 2 serious (1 carotid intramural hematoma, 1 case of needle tract seeding). Intrathyroidal hematomas, dysphagia, tracheal puncture and vasovagal reaction were considered minor. More recently, Park et al.[5] published another systematic review of complications in adults 18-years of age and older. These authors also found very low but variable rates of complications including hematoma formation, neurological symptoms, infection, tracheal puncture and needle-tract implantation (NTI). Only post-FNAC pain was reported as a common complication.

NTI has consistently been reported to be very rare and are most commonly associated with aggressive, poorly differentiated tumors.[3-6] Hayashi et al.[6] evaluated 11,745 patients who underwent FNAC and confirmed that overall rates of NTI are very low (<0.3%) and more likely to occur in patients with aggressive variants. However, these authors stress that NTI should be recognized because the occurrence of NTI following FNAC is likely an indication of the presence of an aggressive neoplasm with increased risk for metastases and death. Thus, one may conclude that there is an overall need for organized, systematic documentation of all adverse events following FNAC performed for any reason.

The literatures cited above made two important points that are relevant to the potential harms of the FHMS thyroid study. 1. Even if the complication rates for FNAC are low, increasing numbers of FNAC performed will lead to increasing total numbers of complications; 2. There is a need for physicians to consider the risk-benefit ratio of FNAC on an individual patient basis before performing the procedure. If FNAC is performed without any proven benefits, the risk for complications will exceed the benefits.

US screening for subclinical thyroid nodules in children inevitably results in increasing numbers of FNAC being performed. The thyroid examination in the FHMS has resulted in FNAC being performed on children and adolescents who, in the absence of screening, either would never undergo the procedure or would undergo FNAC years later for clinically detected nodules amenable to therapy. As discussed in Chapter 2, children with category B nodules are referred for a secondary examination in which experts determine whether FNAC or follow-up is required. Thus, an extremely high number of thyroid biopsies in children have been performed in Fukushima. Increase in FNAC performed for subclinical nodules should be seen as another potentially harmful effect of the thyroid examination in Fukushima and the increasing Japanese enthusiasm for US thyroid screening. One should remember that we do not have adequate data on the numbers of complications of thyroid FNAC in children following mass population screening. This requires a standardized database to record long-term follow-up encompassing patients' personal experiences, including adverse psychologic reactions, and an accurate record of both mild and serious complications.

In summary, one should be concerned that increased FNAC performance owing to US-detected subclinical nodules has the added effect of increasing the total number of complications, both mild and severe. We do not deny that FNAC is a very valuable, minimally invasive diagnostic procedure in some patient groups; however, there must be an attempt to limit FNAC to patients who are likely to benefit from the procedure. When reporting data on FNAC performed on thyroid nodules in children, there should be meticulous follow-up with accurate documentation of the number of adverse effects associated with the procedure. There also should be documentation of how often general anesthesia is required as this adds another very small but finite risk. The only way to minimize the absolute numbers of complications is to limit the absolute numbers of FNAC and attempt to maximize the benefit to risk ratio. All FNAC procedures should be preceded by shared decision making that includes patient, care-giver and a physician who can objectively participate in a balanced discussion of the risks and benefits of FNAC including overdiagnosis.

References
1. Takano T. Natural history of thyroid cancer. ***Endocr J*** 64:237-44, 2017.
2. Hay ID, *et al.* Papillary thyroid carcinoma (PTC) in children and adults: Comparison of initial presentation and long-term postoperative outcome in 4432 patients consecutively treated at the Mayo Clinic during eight decades (1936–2015). ***World J Surg*** 42:329–42, 2018
3. Polyzos SA, Anastasilakis AD. Clinical complications following thyroid fine-needle biopsy: a systematic review. ***Clinic Endocrinol (Oxf)*** 71:157-65, 2009.
4. Cappelli C, *et al.* Complications after fine-needle aspiration cytology; a retrospective study of 7449 consecutive thyroid nodules. ***Br J Oral Maxillofac Surg*** 55:266-9, 2017.
5. Park JY, *et al.* A comprehensive assessment of the harms of fine-needle aspiration biopsy for thyroid nodules: A systematic review. ***Endocrinol Metab (Seoul)*** 38:104-116, 2023.
6. Hayashi T *et al.* Needle tract implantation following fine-needle aspiration of thyroid cancer. ***World J Surg*** 44:378-84, 2020.

Chapter 2
Overview of the thyroid examination in Fukushima

Fukushima Prefecture is located in the northeast of Japan, about 300 km north of Tokyo, with a population of about 2 million in 2011. On March 11, 2011, a magnitude nine earthquake occurred on the northeastern coast of Japan, resulting in tsunamis that caused nearly 20,000 deaths in the coast region. The Fukushima Daiichi nuclear power plant on the Pacific coast lost its core cooling capacity following the tsunami attack, leading to a severe nuclear accident. Large quantities of radioactive material, including radioactive iodine, were released into the environment. Fortunately, the public radiation exposure in Fukushima was much lower than that in Chornobyl due to the lower physical emissions and the plume flow mainly towards the sea, in addition to various measures such as evacuation and monitoring of water and food. No direct radiation health effects, including thyroid cancer, are expected to occur in the future.[1,2] In the aftermath of a major nuclear accident, it is common for residents to be concerned about potential radiation-related health effects, often fueled by media coverage. As a result, health surveys are often conducted to address their health concerns without considering the potential disadvantages of the survey.[2]

In October 2011, six months after the accident, the thyroid ultrasound (US) examination was initiated as part of the Fukushima Health Management Survey (FHMS) in Fukushima Prefecture, although the exposure level in Fukushima caused by the nuclear accident was considered to be much lower than that in Chornobyl. According to the description on the website of the FHMS, the purpose of the thyroid examination was "To address long-term health concerns by understanding the condition of children's thyroid glands, since one of the health problems caused by the Chornobyl nuclear power plant accident was thyroid cancer in childhood caused by internal exposure from radioactive iodine."[3] This chapter is written primarily by two authors, Sanae Midorikawa and Akira Ohtsuru, who were involved in conducting the thyroid examinations in Fukushima Medical University (FMU) and details the inception and implementation of it.

Section 1
How was the thyroid examination started?

The 2011 Fukushima disaster combined a huge earthquake, tsunami, and subsequent nuclear accident. FMU, located 60 km from the Fukushima Daiichi nuclear power plant, was responsible for providing emergent radiation medical care and addressing health problems related to radiation exposure. Ohtsuru *et al.* reported that various additional responses would be required in a nuclear disaster compared to general natural disasters in their review article in the Lancet (Table2-1).[2]

Table 2-1 Required responses in a nuclear disaster
(Created by the authors from ref. 2)

	General response	Special response to nuclear disaster/accident
Disaster onset	Information collection	On-site information gathering
	Search	Launch of off-site center
	Transport	Crisis communication
	Emergency rescue	Evacuation for vulnerable people (Hospital, nursing home, etc.)
	Evacuation	Environmental dose monitoring
	Medical aid station	Iodine prophylaxis
	Shelter management	Radiological screening (food, water, etc)
Initial response phase	Emergency/Disaster medicine	Emergency radiation medicine
	Logistics	Evacuation due to radiological protection
		Sheltering due to radiological protection
		Business continuity plan
	Mental health care	Health surveillance
	Infrastructural development	Individual dose monitoring
Recovery phase		Dose assessment
		Decontamination
		Risk communication
	Preparedness	Nuclear disaster training
Pre-disaster phase	Stockpiles	Evacuation training
	Training	

It is evident that there are numerous issues to address not only in the initial phase but also in the recovery phase following the disaster. Health surveillance after a nuclear accident is deemed necessary in the recovery phase, leading to the implementation of health surveys in Fukushima, called FHMS, such as they were after the Chornobyl and Three Mile Island nuclear accidents. The FHMS, comprising the thyroid examination, individual radiation dose survey, and mental health survey, is conducted by Fukushima Prefecture under contract with FMU.

It is well known that thyroid cancer increased among children following the Chornobyl accident, largely due to internal exposure to milk contaminated with radioactive iodine.[4] A dose-response relationship between thyroid doses and the relative risk of thyroid cancer has been reported.[5] Due to various countermeasures taken to reduce radiation exposure, the thyroid doses of Fukushima residents were deemed much lower than those of Chornobyl residents. However, the residents remained concerned about the possibility of increased thyroid cancer rates. Therefore, the thyroid examination was seen as valuable to the residents if it could confirm that the number of thyroid cancer cases did not increase, even in the context of low radiation doses. The thyroid examination in the FHMS was initiated soon after the accident in October 2011 with the dual purpose of establishing scientific evidence through health surveillance and responding to social concerns by addressing anxiety.[6]

Sometimes, retrospective analysis of actions undertaken with the best of intentions reveals flaws with potentially adverse consequences. The initial part of the thyroid examination consists of mass US screening for cancer. However, there are caveats to consider before the implementation of mass screening. Careful thought must be given as to whether the scientific information of screening program will significantly alleviate subjects' anxieties and whether the benefits of the study outweigh the potential harm. In Fukushima, however, adequate consideration of these caveats had not been given prior to the initiation of mass screening. It was the first time for everyone to experience such a major complex nuclear disaster, so both disaster responders and residents may have felt an obsessive sense of urgency to do something rather than more carefully assess the design of the program prior to its initiation.

The subjects of the thyroid examination were all Fukushima residents aged 18 or younger or *in utero* at the time of the accident. The subjects totaled about 380,000 individuals. As shown in Fig. 2-1, the thyroid examination program consists of two steps: a primary and confirmatory examination.[7] The primary examination is designed to detect the presence of nodules or cysts, using thyroid US for all subjects. Based on the findings, results are divided into Category A (cases not requiring immediate follow-up studies and referred for repeat US in approximately two years) and Category B (cases referred for the confirmatory examination) and sent to the examinees by mail.

Subcategory A1 includes subjects without thyroid nodules or cysts, while subcategory A2 includes subjects with nodules no larger than 5.0 mm and/or cysts no larger than 20.0 mm. Category A cases are not considered medically significant. Examinees with nodules larger than 5.1 mm in diameter are required to undergo a confirmatory examination as Category B. The confirmatory examination includes US, thyroid function testing, serum thyroglobulin, urinary iodine excretion, and if necessary, fine-needle aspiration cytology (FNAC). Following the confirmatory examination, some examinees, including those with suspected thyroid cancer, are referred to a thyroid specialist for further follow-up or treatment.

The first-round examination was intended to assess the prevalence and incidence of thyroid cancer in the absence of radiation exposure effect. Therefore, it was initiated immediately following the accident. Following the first-round examination, the subjects will be examined again every two years until they reach the age of twenty and once every five years thereafter. The thyroid examination is planned to continue for a period of thirty years.

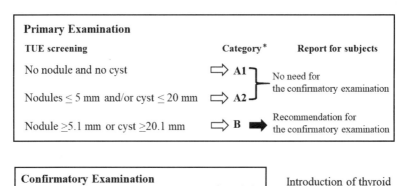

Fig. 2-1 Chart of the thyroid examination (Created by authors from ref. 14)
*A1, A2, and B are the categories in the thyroid ultrasound examination (TUE) report.

Section 2
How the thyroid examination is carried out?

1. Participation in the thyroid examination

Fukushima Prefecture and FMU send notification letters to the subjects of the thyroid examination every two years, which include information on the designated date, time, and location of the examination. Examinations of subjects for primary, secondary, or high school students are performed at the subjects' schools. Thus, the location is given as the school which each student attends. The letter also includes a consent confirmation form and a summary of the thyroid examination, including a brief explanation of purpose and the testing procedure.

In the early phases of the study, the reply form did not include a box for subjects to indicate their refusal to participate. The notification letter simply asked the children to take the examination at the designated location and date. Thus, it did not inform subjects that they were part of a research study, that they could choose not to be examined, nor did it explain the examination's potential harms (risks). It is essential that subjects be provided with sufficient information on the benefits and potential harms of the examination in order to make informed decisions about whether to participate. However, the notification letter in the earlier period did not adequately address these issues. In other words, adequate informed consent was not obtained, even if there was a signature. The problems related to the informed consent of the thyroid examination will also be discussed in the later chapters.

When subjects do not return the consent form to FMU, it is generally assumed that they do not wish to undergo the examination. However, in the early stage of the study, if the subjects' caregivers did not return the consent form, they were contacted by phone or in-person to confirm their refusal to participate. School-aged subjects (elementary, junior high, and high school students) were encouraged to submit the consent form to the school and participate in the examination. For instance, schools sometimes distributed documents urging students to return the unsubmitted consent form as they would any other required materials. Children and their caregivers were also asked by their homeroom or nursing teachers to submit the consent form. This led to the perception that the thyroid examination was essential and mandatory. Under these circumstances, it was very difficult for children to express their desire not to be examined.

2. School examination

The thyroid examination for school-aged subjects is conducted during school classes. FMU and the respective schools coordinate the schedule in advance. Most schools require a full day for the thyroid examination, and the examination is scheduled like other school events, such as sports festivals and school recitals. School teachers and staff are likely to view the examination as an annual school event.

On the day of the examination, medical and official staff visit the school with US equipment. Examination booths are set up in a spacious area, such as a gymnasium, and separated by curtains. Children are brought to the examination site in groups during school classes and examined one by one in the booths. Each examination, which is conducted by skilled medical staff, takes approximately three minutes. It is similar to an assembly line process. Fig. 2-2 shows an image of the thyroid examination at a school.

The examination has achieved a very high participation rate, with over 90% of school-aged children participating, as shown in Table 2-1. This table includes individuals who have moved out of Fukushima Prefecture and is therefore likely to be an underestimation of the actual participation rate within the prefecture, which is likely to be 95% or higher. Few school children have refused to undergo the examination. Those who do not participate in the examination remain in the classroom or accompany others to the examination site but do not undergo the examination themselves.

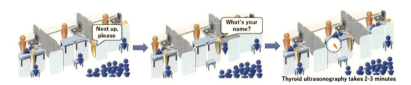

Fig. 2-2 Thyroid examination at school
(Drawing by Manabu Ohishi)

The high participation rate has made it difficult for some children not to participate, even if their parents do not want them to be examined. Some parents have asked the examining physicians to explain to school teachers why they do not want their children to be examined. Children who choose not to participate have faced social pressure, as they are frequently asked by their peers why they are not being examined. These issues were discussed in interviews with school staff at the 40th meeting of the Prefectural

Oversight Committee for the FHMS (POCF).[8]

3. Do subjects undergo the examination because they think it is necessary?

Individuals who have graduated from high school are examined at public facilities or hospitals affiliated with Fukushima Prefecture. The participation rate for this group drops sharply in the second round to 10-20%, as shown in Table 2-2.[9] This trend becomes more pronounced in the third round. This decrease in the participation rate suggests that subjects who have graduated from high school no longer feel pressured to participate. If subjects had been truly concerned about the health effects of radiation, it is unlikely that such concerns would rapidly diminish after graduation from high school.

Table 2-2 Participation rate by age group (%)

Age	1st round	2nd round	3rd round
0	85.3		
1	85		
2	80.3	69.1	
3	81.4	69.1	
4	83.3	71.4	50.6
5	84.3	71.8	53.2
6	95	92	88.6
7	95.7	92.8	89.5
8	95.7	93.1	90.2
9	95.9	93.6	90.3
10	95.9	93.8	90.6
11	96.1	93.8	90.6
12	96	92.7	89.1
13	95.2	91.7	88.2
14	94.3	91.2	87.6
15	75.3	86.2	80
16	74	86.4	80.5
17	67.6	79.2	75.3
18	52.8	33.5	22.5
19	44	28.4	18.2
20	30.5	24.4	14.9
21		21.3	14.3
22		16.1	11.8
23			
24			9.9
total	81.7	71	61.3

The participation rate for preschool children, whose caregivers may have a strong concern about the effects of radiation, also drops to 50% in the third round. In contrast, the participation rate of school-aged children remains consistently at around 80-90%. The fact that only the participation rate for school-aged children remains high suggests that many of these children may be undergoing the thyroid examination simply because it is conducted during school classes rather than due to a belief that it is necessary. In other words, the examination system in school does not adequately ensure voluntary participation.[10]

To determine the reasons why subjects are undertaking the examination after graduating from high school, Midorikawa *et al.* conducted face-to-face interviews with examinees at public facilities between February and March 2018 (reported at the 1st International Symposium of the Radiation Medical Science Center for the Fukushima Health Management Survey 2019). Most of them were college students or adults. As shown in Table 2-3, the most common reason given for participating was "I thought I had to take the examination," followed by recommendations from family members. Some examinees who indicated that they were "worried about the health effects of radiation" or "worried about thyroid disease" had previously been diagnosed with US findings, such as cysts or nodules, during the screening process.

One examinee who was interviewed stated, "I had undergone the examination at school before, so I thought I had to take the examination." Another examinee said, "I did not reply to the first notification letter for the thyroid examination. However, I felt I had to take the examination when I received the reminder postcard for non-examinees." This response suggests that the reminder postcard may persuade those who do not respond to the initial notification letter to participate in the examination. Thus, even the examinees at public facilities, usually considered voluntary participants, are likely to regard the thyroid examination as mandatory. Furthermore, such opinions were expressed by the parents of the subjects and by a subject herself at symposiums held by the Japan Consortium of Juvenile Thyroid Cancer (JCJTC).[11, 12]

Table 2-3 Reasons for participation

They thought they had to take the examination	35%
Their family recommended the examination	28%
Worried about the health effects of radiation	16%
Worried about thyroid disease	7%
Others	15%

4. Problems with how to explain the results

The results of the thyroid examination conducted at each school, public facility, and contracted hospital, including ultrasound images and reports written by an examiner (either a doctor or clinical laboratory technician), are collected at FMU. These results are then reviewed by the Judgment Committee, comprising several thyroid specialists, who check the images and reports and classify the confirmed results (as shown in Fig. 2-1). The results are then mailed to the individual in written form approximately 2-3 months later.

During the first four years of the thyroid examination, the examiners were not permitted to explain the results to the examinees or their caregivers on-site. This led to anxiety among the examinees and their caregivers, who were left uncertain about their results. In routine clinical practice, a physician would explain the results of a US examination in person. However, in Fukushima, this was not possible due to the large number of participants and the fact that, in Japan, clinical laboratory technicians are not allowed to explain the results.

The results of the thyroid examination are summarized by FMU and reported to the POCF approximately every three months as survey results. The progress of the examination, participation rate, and results (including the number of cancers detected) are publicly reported and discussed among the experts at the POCF meeting. These experts provide comments on the FHMS methods and results, including the thyroid examination, to the prefecture and the media. The mass media has reported the survey results and the experts' comments in newspapers, on TV programs, and on the internet. As described in later chapters, many of these reports have caused public anxiety and have often presented biased opinions rather than providing objective reporting.

5. The subjects of the thyroid examination were not informed of the purpose, benefits, or potential harms (risks) of the study

When implementing the thyroid examination, the FHMS leadership must educate physicians, examinees, and the general public to prevent harmful misconceptions. All must understand that: 1. Thyroid nodules and cysts are common US findings in all populations regardless of history of radiation exposure; 2. Finding a thyroid nodule, cyst, or cancer by US does not mean that these lesions are related to radiation; 3. Most US-detected thyroid nodules are benign and unlikely to cause harm; 4. Even most malignant nodules detected by high-sensitive US screening in asymptomatic people are unlikely to cause harm.

Furthermore, before anyone is enlisted in the thyroid US examination (TUE), the subject should be informed of the following facts: 1. The radiation dose in Fukushima was not high enough to be a risk factor for thyroid cancer; 2. A TUE can lead to the detection of innocuous lesions, including cancer overdiagnosis; 3. The examination is not mandatory and there will be no inconvenience nor punishment for refusal to participate; 4. The thyroid examination is being done as a research project to gain information about thyroid nodules in Japan and may not benefit one's health; 5. The main harm of the TUE is cancer overdiagnosis/overtreatment and associated psychosocial disadvantages.

However, at that time, parents in Fukushima were very worried about their children's health, especially thyroid cancer, after seeing the Chornobyl nuclear accident reported in the media as a comparison. The thyroid examination in Fukushima was implemented in a hurried fashion owing to the need to rapidly address residents' concerns about the health effects of radiation, including the risk of thyroid cancer. Even though parents of children who participated in the study experienced some anxiety, time was not taken to carefully explain the purpose of the study, nor were the benefits, risks, and right to refuse participation to subjects or their caregivers. Also, it was a few years after the initiation of the thyroid examination when the serious overdiagnosis consequences of US thyroid screening in South Korea were reported.[13] Thus, the possibility of overdiagnosis was not considered a serious matter or was not discussed before the initiation of the thyroid examination.

Midorikawa and Ohtsuru had conducted classes on the thyroid examination in some elementary, junior high, and senior high schools on request.[14] The children were familiar with the location of the thyroid gland because they were subjects of the thyroid examination; however, very few understood why the thyroid examination was being conducted. The residents of Fukushima, including caregivers of the screening subjects, have little knowledge about the thyroid examination, and a questionnaire study revealed that less than 20% of the subjects understand the potential harm of the examination.[15]

The initial purpose of the thyroid examination was to monitor the children's health after the nuclear accident. At some point, the purpose was expanded to include a survey to "investigate the health effects of radiation." However, no opportunity has been provided to explain this addition to the residents.

Despite discussions about the necessity of explaining the harm of thyroid cancer screening at the POCF, no opportunity has been provided to explain it to the subjects in an easily understandable manner. The thyroid examination is currently in its sixth round, and the subjects are becoming accustomed to participating in the thyroid examination without knowing its significance or the harm of overdiagnosis.

Although it may take a significant amount of time, it is important for the examiners to speak with the residents face to face and help them understand the nature of the thyroid examination based on scientific findings. In addition, in order to mitigate the potential harms of the examination and prevent pressure to participate, consideration should be given to removing the US screening program from a school-based setting and using an opt-in rather than opt-out consent form.[15] Consideration should also be given to discontinuing the examination for all except voluntary participants who are fully aware of the risks and wish to participate for the sake of scientific research.

Section 3
Summary of the results of the thyroid examination during 2011-2023

Table 2-4 summarizes the five rounds of thyroid cancer screening and thyroid cancer screening of 25 and 30-year-olds during the past 12 years in the thyroid examination of the FHMS.[16] The data were updated on February 2, 2024, at the 50th meeting of the POCF. In primary screening, the first round was conducted from fiscal years 2011 to 2013, the second round was from fiscal years 2014 to 2015, the third round was from fiscal years 2016 to 2017, the fourth round was from fiscal years 2018 to 2019, and the fifth round was from fiscal years 2020 to 2022. The results of examinations for 25- and 30-year-olds are shown in the two columns at the bottom. As mentioned above, as the number of generations without school examinations increased, the participation rate decreased.

Table 2-4 Summary of the results of the thyroid examination from 2011 to 2023

rounds	primary examination					confirmatory examination	
	participation		category			number of detected thyroid cancer	*corrected detection rate (/10^5)
	n	Rate (%)	A1 (%)	A2 (%)	B (%)		
1st(2011-13)	300,472	81.7	51.5	47.8	0.8	116	42.3
2nd (2014-15)	270,552	71.0	40.2	59.0	0.8	71	31.9
3rd (2016-17)	217,922	64.7	35.1	64.2	0.7	31	20.0
4th (2018-19)	183,410	62.3	33.6	65.6	0.8	39	29.2
5th (2020-22)	113,941	45.0	28.8	70.0	1.2	43	50.4
25 years-old	11,867	9.2	42.5	52.0	5.5	23	234.4
30 years-old	1,571	6.9	44.6	46.9	8.6	5	444.1

*Corrected thyroid cancer detection rate per 100,000 examinees in the primary examination is calculated by correcting the rates of participation and confirmed results in the confirmatory examination.

Regarding the results of the primary examination, the A1 category accounted for 28.8% to 51.5%, the A2 category accounted for 46.9% to 70.0%, and the B category accounted for 0.7% to 8.6%. The A2 category was mostly cysts and some nodules. The number of B category cases increased with age, and most cases were nodules. These results caused great confusion because there was little experience with this screening, which uses sophisticated US equipment, and because it was started after the nuclear accident. More details on this will be given in Chapter 3.

In the confirmatory examination, malignant or suspicious malignant cases were detected using FNAC. In the first round, 116 cases were diagnosed, with 71 cases in the second round, 31 in the third round, 39 in the fourth round, 43 cases in the fifth round, and 23 cases and 5 cases in the examination of 25- and 30-year-olds. The confirmatory examination in the fifth round and the examination of 25- and 30-year-olds are ongoing. The most common pathological type among surgical cases was papillary thyroid cancer (PTC).

In the rightmost column, the thyroid cancer detection rate per 100,000 examinees in the primary examination is calculated by correcting the rates of participation and confirmed results in the confirmatory examination. These rates were not adjusted for age, sex, number of screenings, intervals between screenings, and other factors from cancer registries. The thyroid cancer incidence from 2001 to 2010 by the Japanese national cancer registry indicates 0.0 for 0-9 years of age, 0.2 for 10-14 years of age, 0.7 for 15-19 years of age, 2.0 for 20-24 years of age, 2.8 for 25-29 years of age per 10^5 people. These data on cancer registry incidence are thought to be almost non-screening conditions. Although a direct comparison is not possible, there is considerable that the TUE screening resulted in marked increased cancer detection and potential overdiagnosis more than ten times greater.[17] Please see Chapter 1 and the following chapters to find out how these results can be explained, what they mean for the participants, their families, and their communities, and how FMU, Fukushima Prefecture, and the academic community have responded.

References
1. UNSCEAR. Vienna, Austria: UNSCEAR 2020/2021 report volume II. [internet, cited 2024 July 15] Available from: https://www.unscear.org/unscear/en/publications/2020_2021_2.html.
2. Ohtsuru A, *et al.* Nuclear disasters and health: lessons learned, challenges, and proposals. ***Lancet*** 386:489-97, 2015.

3. Radiation Medical Science Center for the Fukushima Health Management Survey. Fukushima, Japan: Thyroid Ultrasound Examination. [internet, cited 2024 July 15] Available from: https://fhms.jp/en/fhms/thyroid/.
4. Drozdovitch V. Radiation exposure to the thyroid after the Chernobyl accident. *Front Endocrinol (Lausanne)* 11:569041, 2021.
5. Brenner AV, *et al.* I-131 dose response for incident thyroid cancers in Ukraine related to the Chornobyl accident. *Environ Health Perspect* 119:933-9, 2011.
6. Yasumura S, *et al.* Study protocol for the Fukushima Health Management Survey. *J Epidemiol* 22:375-83, 2012.
7. Suzuki S, *et al.* The protocol and preliminary baseline survey results of the thyroid ultrasound examination in Fukushima *Endocr J* 63:315-21, 2016.
8. Fukushima Prefecture. Fukushima, Japan: The results of the survey on the current status of the thyroid examination at schools (in Japanese). [internet, cited 2024 July 15] Available from: https://www.pref.fukushima.lg.jp/uploaded/attachment/422936.pdf.
9. Fukushima Prefecture. Fukushima, Japan: The results of each examination (in Japanese). [internet, cited 2024 July 15] Available from: https://www.pref.fukushima.lg.jp/uploaded/attachment/389708.pdf.
10. Midorikawa S, Ohtsuru A. Disaster-zone research: make participation voluntary. *Nature* 579:193, 2020.
11. Japan Consortium of Juvenile Thyroid Cancer. Japan: Thyroid Cancer Overdiagnosis: Voice from Fukushima 2. [internet, cited 2024 July 15] Available from: https://www.youtube.com/watch?v=NvAvvvbODW4.
12. Japan Consortium of Juvenile Thyroid Cancer. Japan: Thyroid Cancer Overdiagnosis 3-3: Opinion of an examinee. [internet, cited 2024 July 15] Available from: https://www.youtube.com/watch?v=7WsdED9LY0I.
13. Ahn HS, *et al.* Korea's thyroid-cancer "epidemic"--screening and overdiagnosis. *N Engl J Med* 371:1765-7, 2014.
14. Midorikawa S, *et al.* Psychosocial issues related to thyroid examination after a radiation disaster. *Asia Pac J Pub Health* 29:63S-73S, 2017.
15. Midorikawa S, Ohtsuru A. Young people's perspectives of thyroid cancer screening and its harms after the nuclear accident in Fukushima Prefecture: a questionnaire survey indicating opt-out screening strategy of the thyroid examination as an ethical issue. *BMC Cancer* 22:235, 2022.
16. Fukushima Prefecture. Fukushima, Japan: Materials from the 50th meeting of the Prefectural Oversight Committee for the FHMS (in Japanese). [internet, cited 2024

July 15] Available from: https://www.pref.fukushima.lg.jp/sec/21045b/kenkocyosa-kentoiinkai-50.html.
17. Ohtsuru A, *et al.* Incidence of thyroid cancer among children and young adults in Fukushima, Japan, screened with 2 rounds of ultrasonography within 5 years of the 2011 Fukushima Daiichi Nuclear Power Station accident. ***JAMA Otolaryngol Head Neck Surg*** 145:4–11, 2019.

Chapter 3
What happened to the children after taking the thyroid examination?

The purpose of the thyroid examination in Fukushima was to monitor with care (in a Japanese word, "yorisou") the health of children in Fukushima whose families were concerned about the health effects of radiation exposure. It was in retrospect, too optimistic, but it was hoped that this monitoring and support would bring peace of mind, confidence, and happiness to the children and their families. Some of the authors (Midorikawa and Ohtsuru) who have previously participated in this program know well that staff and colleagues involved have been working diligently to achieve these goals. Just as it is necessary for medical practitioners to reflect on their medical practice from the patient's point of view, it is also important to know how this ultrasound (US) screening examination affected the subject and their family. In this chapter, the authors describe the feelings of the children and residents in Fukushima during this time and encourage readers to consider how they might feel in a similar situation.

Section 1
The confusion caused by the category "A2"

As described in Chapter 2, the examination results are categorized into A1, A2, and B. These categories are unfamiliar to the subjects and their parents. They were specifically designed for this thyroid US examination (TUE). A reporting letter of the result is mailed to the examinees. An example of the letter is, "Your US finding shows a small cyst. This is category A2. There is nothing wrong with it." The reporting letter includes a brief explanation of cysts and nodules, but this explanation was insufficient to alleviate their concerns. Approximately half, more than 150,000 of the examinees had cysts that were classified as A2.[1] These cysts rarely have any pathological significance and do not indicate the presence of disease. However, the subjects and their families had many questions, such as: What is a cyst? Can it be left untreated? Can it turn into cancer? Was it caused by radiation? As a result, the call center of Fukushima Medical University (FMU) received many inquiries daily. The TUE caused increased anxiety because of this inappropriate way of delivering results.[2]

The TUE also led to feelings of guilt in caregivers, particularly mothers, who believed the results were related to their actions immediately after the nuclear accident.[2] They wondered if their children's cysts were caused by their decision not to evacuate, by feeding them food from Fukushima, or by allowing them to play outside. Some very anxious individuals even evacuated from Fukushima after receiving the examination results.

The thyroid examination is done by US and is used to detect the presence of thyroid lesions (cysts or solid nodules). US evaluation cannot estimate individual radiation doses, nor can it assess for radiation effects on the thyroid gland. It is an epidemiological survey of the population and cannot determine the relationship between US findings and radiation exposure on an individual basis. The residents were not fully informed of this, leading them to link the US findings to the effects of radiation exposure and experience self-condemnation. This self-condemnation can lead to stigma (branding or prejudice) and self-stigma (prejudice against oneself) due to presumed radiation exposure.[2,3]

This confusion surrounding category A2 in the TUE results became a social issue known as the "A2 problem" in Fukushima. For example, a newspaper headline stated, "Is the result of category A2 OK?" Many examinees requested more information about the results of their examination, including US photographs. The explanation from FMU that there was no problem with cysts was not sufficient to comfort or reassure patients.

To address this confusion, the Ministry of the Environment conducted a project called the "3-prefecture examination," in which children of almost the same age as those in the Fukushima Health Management Survey (FHMS) in Aomori, Yamanashi, and Nagasaki prefectures away from Fukushima were examined in the same way. The results showed that children in these prefectures had high rates of cysts, similar to those found in Fukushima.[4]

This report indeed provided some relief about the A2 problem, and afterward, it was not so difficult to explain that A2 is no problem. However, it may have also given the impression that mass screenings are acceptable methods to address anxiety related to a nuclear plant accident. Retrospectively, it may, in fact, be unethical to screen in other prefectures to explain or reassure that overdiagnosis is common for cysts and nodules in TUE mass screening. Midorikawa and Ohtsuru regret the implementation of the Fukushima TUE project. They believe that there are better methods to assuage fears, such as carefully explaining the health risks of radiation to the residents. Education and discussion should have been used in place of this problematic research.

Section 2
What happened to the children who were diagnosed to have a thyroid nodule?

The result of category B in the TUE is notified by a letter stating, "You have a nodule. You will receive a separate notice letter for the detailed examination." Those who receive this result often become very anxious. In the first round of the examination alone, over 2,000 children received a category B result.[1] Actually, most thyroid nodules were benign, with at least 90% not requiring a detailed examination or treatment. However, before the detailed examination, notified individuals may worry that they have cancer or have been harmed by radiation. This can be a psychological burden.[3] The majority of the children who received a category B result did not actually have cancer. This means that category B had a high rate of "false positives" in cancer screening terminology. In order to increase the positive predictive value of screening (the probability that people with positive tests really have cancer) and to reduce harm, one needs to minimize false positives as much as possible. However, if one assumes that most of TUE-detected true positives are self-limiting or indolent neoplasms, decreasing the rate of false positives will not solve the problem of overdiagnosis.

Most people are relieved when the detailed examination shows that they have a benign nodule that does not require treatment. However, they may still be concerned about whether the nodule can be left as it is and may wish to have a follow-up observation. Even if the nodule is not cancer, these examinees and their caregivers may face uncertainty about whether they can stop follow-up observation, how long they should continue surveillance, and whether radiation caused the nodule. Those who no longer need follow-up observation may still worry. For example, if they catch a cold and have enlarged lymph nodes in their neck, they may suspect that their thyroid nodule is causing the neck swelling. In this way, detection of even a benign, incidental thyroid nodule can have harmful effects.

It is well known that the number of people with thyroid nodules increases with age.[5] In adults, 10-20% of people have thyroid nodules, which would be classified as category B in the Fukushima examination. As shown in Table 2-4 in Chapter 2, the percentage of category B in TUE for 25-year-olds is 5.4% and 8.5% for 30-year-olds compared to 0.7% to 1.2% for school-aged children, main subjects in the first to fifth rounds. This means that the number of false positives from the screening will increase as the thyroid examination continues. At a meeting of the Prefectural Oversight Committee of the Fukushima Health Management Survey (POCF), an epidemiologist pointed out these concerns, but no measures have been taken since then.[6]

Section 3
Impact of publicizing the examination results

The survey results of the thyroid examination are reported by FMU to the POCF approximately once every three months in early days. The residents are informed of the overall results through media coverage of the POCF meeting reports. As a result, information focusing on the number of thyroid cancer cases that increased due to the examination is widely disseminated through television and newspapers every three months.

In Japan, municipalities conduct five types of cancer screening every year or every two years, but their results are not widely publicized by the media. The widespread reporting of thyroid cancer screening in response to the nuclear accident may have led many people to believe that radiation has had an adverse effect on the residents of Fukushima. The POCF ultimately concluded that the thyroid cancers discovered in both the first and second rounds of thyroid examinations were not likely to be caused by radiation exposure.[7,8] However, this conclusion was not widely communicated to the public.

If the purpose of the thyroid examination is to monitor children's individual health, its results should be communicated privately and confidentially to participants and their caregivers. However, when these results are used in a survey to assess the health effects of radiation, comprehensive results of the thyroid examination are made public. Publicization of the rate of thyroid cancer detection could cause concern in people who previously believed that the low levels of radiation exposure in Fukushima posed little risk. These individuals may then overestimate the risk of thyroid cancer due to radiation exposure, leading to increased anxiety and fears. Thus, instead of assuaging fears, the results of the thyroid examination have had the unintended consequences of deepening concerns and increasing risk perception about radiation exposure.[3, 9]

Furthermore, many people outside of Fukushima or not closely following the Fukushima nuclear power plant accident believe that thyroid cancer is increasing in Fukushima due to radiation. The widespread misunderstanding throughout Japan and worldwide that thyroid cancer is increasing in Fukushima due to radiation has been caused by the thyroid examination itself. In fact, a questionnaire survey found that approximately 40% of Fukushima residents in the evacuation area and over 50% of Tokyo residents believe that cancer will increase in Fukushima due to radiation exposure.[10] This shows that residents in Tokyo have a higher risk perception of the effect of radiation. Ironically, residents from regions remote from Fukushima seem less apt to accept the scientific evidence that the radiation released from Fukushima imposed little or no risk to the local population. When the media promotes biased perceptions not supported by scientific evidence, significant damage is done to society.

Section 4
Impact of the results on examinees' sense of security and misunderstanding

Initially, the results of the thyroid examination were not explained to each examinee immediately following the TUE for the reasons described in Chapter 2. This lack of explanation contributed to increased anxiety among the residents. Therefore, when Midorikawa and Ohtsuru took on leadership roles in the thyroid examination, they implemented a system to provide face-to-face explanations of the results to examinees immediately after the TUE. Doctors show the US images to the examinees and their caregivers and explain the meaning of the findings at the examination venues.

This immediate post-examination private counseling, including US image presentation, was provided on a trial basis starting in October 2014, was officially implemented in April 2015, and continues to this day even after leadership changes. This enables doctors to discuss the significance of cysts or nodules with examinees while showing them the US images. Many examinees and caregivers have stated that their anxiety was relieved after receiving this counseling, compared to their previous examinations[3, 9]. However, onsite counseling is not in place for school examinations. It means that most school-age subjects (ages 6-18) and their parents were not available for onsite counseling. Onsite counseling has also allowed medical staff to answer questions about the relationship between thyroid nodules and radiation exposure. However, few people asked such questions, even those with health concerns after the nuclear accident. This may be the limit of the onsite counseling.

Unexpectedly, the reassurance provided by the explanation led to new misconceptions. Participants and their caregivers mistakenly understood that the absence of abnormal findings meant that participants had not been adversely affected by radiation. The TUE can only determine the presence or absence of thyroid lesions. It cannot determine whether the lesions are related to radiation exposure. Nor can the examination predict whether there have been or will be adverse radiation effects on the individual. Only long-term epidemiological analysis can examine the effects of radiation on the population.

Section 5
What happened when the thyroid examination found cancer?

As mentioned in previous sections, the detection of thyroid nodules or cysts alone causes concern that these lesions, although common and benign, are indications of radiation effect. When the TUE and follow-up detects thyroid cancer in children or young adults, both the examinees and their caretakers often become even more distressed. In Fukushima, those diagnosed with thyroid cancer tend to believe radiation exposure is the cause.

There are two reasons for this misconception. The Fukushima thyroid cancers were detected in children shortly after the Fukushima accident during the thyroid examination, which was initiated following the nuclear accident. Everyone has a tendency to think that there is only one cause of cancer, so it is not unreasonable for the residents to think that radiation from the nuclear accident is the cause. Second, it is widely known and scientifically accepted that there was a radiation-related increase in pediatric thyroid cancer following the Chornobyl nuclear accident. It is no wonder that residents are tempted to think of Chornobyl as the same phenomenon rather than considering the difference.

Fukushima residents have not been adequately informed that: 1. The situation in Chornobyl was quite different from that in Fukushima; 2. The FHMS detected cancers too soon after the accident to have been related to radiation in the first and second rounds; 3. We now know that subclinical or self-limiting papillary thyroid carcinomas (PTC) are common findings in children without radiation exposure. It is likely that some of the childhood PTC found in Chornobyl screening were also spontaneous rather than radiation-related.

Dealing with the aftermath of a nuclear plant accident, whether radiation levels released are high (as in Chornobyl) or low (as in Fukushima), is a Herculean task.[11] While prompt information disclosure is generally desired immediately following the accident, there is confusion, premature release of information that may not be accurate, and rampant fear. There is general knowledge that radiation exposure can lead to cancer, and after a nuclear plant accident, people assume that any cancers found after the accident are related to radiation.

What the general public does not understand is that: chronic exposure to low dose radiation is common in the environment globally; radiation-related cancers require about 5 years to develop;[12, 13] and incidental thyroid carcinomas are common incidental autopsy findings in adults who die of other cases. Now we also know that subclinical, self-limiting PTC are common findings in children who undergo thyroid US screening. However, most people cannot be convinced, and they may even wonder, "If not caused by radiation exposure, then what is it?" and become even more distressed.

There have been serious psychosocial consequences of the Fukushima thyroid examination program. These include caregiver guilt and self-condemnation, discrimination against- or stigmatization of examinees, and fear that children's bodies have been damaged by radiation.[3, 9, 14] The psychological and social disadvantages are enhanced by the belief that the cancer was caused by radiation exposure. For example, the concern or worry that radiation exposure caused thyroid cancer may lead to regretting one's actions at the time (self-condemnation) or feeling as if one's body has been injured by radiation. Some people may be troubled by the misconception that radiation-induced cancer is more malignant. In addition, the scientifically incorrect idea that cancer in Fukushima is caused by radiation exposure may lead to social discrimination.[3, 9, 14] When there are repeated media reports that thyroid cancer is increasing among children and young people in Fukushima, more and more residents may become concerned that they may have thyroid cancer, in addition to concerns about radiation exposure.

In addition to these socio-psychological effects, the socialization of Raffle and Gray's "popularity paradox" has occurred in Fukushima because detecting early, overdiagnosed PTC convinces people that lives are being saved.[15] The number of thyroid US examinations increased rapidly in Fukushima and neighboring prefectures after the nuclear accident.

References

1. Shimura H, et al. Findings of thyroid ultrasound examination within 3 years after the Fukushima nuclear power plant accident: The Fukushima Health Management Survey. *J Clin Endocrinol Metab* 103:861-9, 2018.
2. Midorikawa S, et al. After Fukushima: addressing anxiety. *Science* 352: 666-7, 2016.
3. Midorikawa S, et al. Psychosocial issues related to thyroid examination after a radiation disaster. *Asia Pac J Public Health* 29 (2S):63S-73S, 2017.
4. Hayashida N, et al. Thyroid ultrasound findings in children from three Japanese prefectures: Aomori, Yamanashi and Nagasaki. *PLoS One* 8(12):e83220, 2013.
5. Shimura H, et al. Epidemiology of thyroid tumor (detection rate of incident tumor, incidence, risk factor, and prognosis in Japan). *Endocrinology, Diabetology and Metabolism* 29: 179-85, 2009 (in Japanese).
6. Fukushima Prefecture. Fukushima, Japan: The proceeding of the 35th Fukushima Prefectural Oversight Committee Meeting (in Japanese) . [internet, cited 2024 July 15] Available from: https://www.pref.fukushima.lg.jp/uploaded/attachment/344571.pdf.
7. Fukushima Prefecture. Fukushima, Japan: Interim report of the Fukushima Health Management Survey (in Japanese). [internet, cited 2024 July 15] Available from: https://www.pref.fukushima.lg.jp/uploaded/attachment/158522.pdf.
8. Fukushima Prefecture Fukushima, Japan: Summary on the results of the full scale thyroid examination (second round) (in Japanese). [internet, cited 2024 July 15] Available from: https://www.pref.fukushima.lg.jp/uploaded/attachment/339634.pdf.
9. Midorikawa S, et al. Psychosocial impact on the thyroid examination of the Fukushima Health Management Survey. In: Thyroid cancer and nuclear accidents: long-term aftereffects of Chernobyl and Fukushima (1st ed.). Academic Press, pp.165-73, 2017.
10. Mitsubishi Research Institute. Tokyo, Japan: With the Tokyo Olympics approaching, it is necessary to reaffirm awareness of the state of reconstruction in Fukushima

Prefecture and the health effects of radiation (Part 1) (in Japanese). [internet, cited 2024 July 15]
Available from: https://www.mri.co.jp/opinion/column/trend/trend_20171114.html.
11. Ohtsuru A, et al. Nuclear disasters and health: lessons learned, challenges, and proposals *Lancet* 386:489-97, 2015.
12. Thomas G, Yamashita S. Thirty years after Chernobyl and 5 after Fukushima-what have we learnt and what do we still need to know? In: Thyroid cancer and nuclear accidents: Long-term aftereffects of Chernobyl and Fukushima (1st ed.). Academic Press, pp. xv-xxiv, 2017.
13. Boice JD. From Chernobyl and beyond-a focus on thyroid cancer. In: Thyroid cancer and nuclear accidents: Long-term aftereffects of Chernobyl and Fukushima (1st ed.). Academic Press, pp.21-32, 2017.
14. Midorikawa S, et al. Harm of overdiagnosis or extremely early diagnosis behind trends in pediatric thyroid cancer. *Cancer*, 125:4108-9, 2019.
15. Raffle AE, Gray JAM. Popularity paradox. In: Screening: Evidence and Practice. Oxford University Press, p.68, 2007.

Chapter 4
Overdiagnosis of thyroid cancer in Fukushima: How did it start and expand?

This chapter focuses on how the Fukushima Health Management Survey (FHMS) was started; how the detection of many unexpected thyroid cancers raised concerns about overdiagnosis and its harms; and how these concerns led to disputes between the FHMS leadership and others involved in the thyroid examination program. The chapter's goal is to become an essential resource for understanding the causes of the thyroid cancer overdiagnosis problem in Fukushima.

Section 1
The origins of a huge thyroid cancer screening program

The basic plan of the FHMS was announced in September 2011. Many Japanese experts were surprised that such a massive project would be launched. After the nuclear plant accident, appropriate measures were taken to prevent radiation exposure of Fukushima residents such as the restriction on milk shipments. The radiation exposure dose in Fukushima was, therefore, estimated to be much less than in Chornobyl. As a result, it was believed that the exposure dose was not at a sufficiently high level to increase the risk of thyroid cancer.[1] Investigators did not expect to find the increased number of thyroid cancers revealed by the baseline thyroid ultrasound (US) examination.

As partly stated in Chapter 3, the purpose of the thyroid examination was "to monitor with caring (*yorisou*)." This phrase is ambiguous but can be interpreted to mean that the thyroid examination was intended to alleviate anxiety among Fukushima residents. It is clear, however, that the project's purpose was not to improve children's health because the FHMS had no data to suggest that children would benefit from early detection of thyroid cancer by US.

As described in Chapter 1, after the Chornobyl nuclear power plant disaster, Japanese specialists were recruited to help orchestrate and implement a screening program for thyroid cancer. The Japanese consultants were welcomed ceremoniously in Red Square, Moscow.[2] The Japanese led health screening program contributed valuable information regarding the effect of high levels of ^{131}I exposure on children's thyroid glands and the need for further research. There is now no doubt that very young children have an increased risk for papillary thyroid carcinoma (PTC) after exposure to high levels of radiation. However, at that time, the following were not known to investigators: radiation-induced thyroid cancers are not more aggressive than spontaneous cancers; small, subclinical PTC are common in childhood; most PTC are either indolent or self-limiting and rarely cause death; and screening for thyroid cancer can cause psychosocial harms owing to overdiagnosis and diagnosis-too-early. The positive contributions of the Chornobyl screening program were known, but its harms were not recognized.

Therefore, it is easy to imagine that the perceived success of the Chornobyl experience would lead to support for launching a similar project in Fukushima. Many specialists involved in the project in Chornobyl also took part in planning the FHMS. Thus, there is reason to believe that the Fukushima thyroid examination program was intended to provide the same standard of care as was provided to the residents around Chornobyl so that Fukushima residents would not feel neglected.

The following remark by an expert is recorded in the minutes of the prefectural meeting discussing the measures after the nuclear accident.[3] "The data obtained by the FHMS will be of value in the event of proceedings related to a nuclear plant accident in the future." This explains the reason why *all* children were enrolled. The thyroid examination in Fukushima was started as an *epidemiological* study to meet political and social demands rather than a medically-oriented project aimed at improving the health of Fukushima children.

Section 2
The FHMS leadership had high hopes, but the results were not what they expected

The thyroid examination was started in late 2011. In the related Japanese academic societies, there was widespread elation and enthusiasm for starting a vast, groundbreaking project which had not been done before in any other part of the world. Thyroid experts at the time believed in the classical multistep carcinogenesis theory of the natural history of thyroid cancer. This theory espouses the idea that well differentiated thyroid cancers (papillary and follicular) are derived from adult (differentiated) follicular cells and can progress to poorly differentiated/anaplastic aggressive carcinomas due to the accumulation of genetic alterations.[4] Progression to poorly differentiated or anaplastic carcinoma usually occurs in older adults.

If this is true, one should not expect to detect thyroid cancer in childhood; therefore, no matter how careful the thyroid US screening is, the number of thyroid cancers detected in Fukushima should be very small given the population's low dose of radiation exposure and the very short interval between the power plant accident and initiation of the thyroid examination. The plan that the FHMS submitted to the ethics committee of Fukushima Medical University stated that thyroid US is harmless, and thyroid cancer in children is rare. The concept of overdiagnosis was not well known at the time, and the harms of screening was not recognized.

The leadership of the thyroid US examination (TUE) had expected that that their large-scale survey would detect only a small number of childhood thyroid cancer and thus would reassure Fukushima residents that there would be no increase in thyroid cancer as occurred in Chornobyl.

However, their optimism proved to be misplaced since the baseline TUE revealed

113 cases of suspected cancer and 98 cases of thyroid cancer proven by postoperative pathology.[5] The baseline TUE survey was initiated in 2011 in the most heavily contaminated areas in Fukushima followed by screening in areas with intermediate and low levels contamination in fiscal years 2012 and 2013, respectively. Surprisingly, there was little difference in the percentages of thyroid cancer detected in the high, intermediate and low contamination areas.[5] These results were transmitted to the public via the media, and rumors were disseminated that thyroid cancer in children was increasing due to radiation. Ironically, although the government's intention was to use the thyroid examination to eliminate Fukushima residents' anxiety, the examination, in fact, led to increased anxiety and social turmoil.

Section 3
Controversy regarding thyroid cancer, is it radiation-induced or caused by screening effect?

The finding of thyroid cancer or suspected thyroid cancer in over 100 children during the baseline thyroid examination sparked debate regarding whether results reflected increased thyroid cancer owing to radiation exposure or high resolution US screening. Some researchers believe that radiation likely contributed to thyroid cancers detected in Fukushima prefecture zones with high radiation contamination. They reject the idea that intense US screening was detecting spontaneous, subclinical cancers in Fukushima.[6] However, many consider this concept flawed and potentially harmful.[7] It was clear, based on finding PTC similarly even in the minimally contaminated Aizu region of Fukushima, that radiation was not causing Fukushima's thyroid cancers. Unreasonable attribution of thyroid cancer to minimal doses of radiation exposure, not dissimilar to ambient environmental radiation, can cause widespread fear lasting for decades and may encourage the implementation of future screening programs following nuclear accidents as a kind of political driver.

Section 4
The results of the second round confirmed the outbreak of overdiagnosis

The results of the first round examination indicated that in Japanese children, there is a sizable reservoir of subclinical PTC which are susceptible to detection by high resolution US, thus fulfilling Black and Welch's prerequisites for overdiagnosis.[8] This unexpected finding, along with new ideas regarding the natural history of thyroid cancer, should have been a warning sign for potential overdiagnosis.[9] Most cancers develop in middle-aged to elderly adults and are believed to become invasive and increasingly aggressive owing to a multistep series of genetic mutations and epigenetic alterations.[4] We now know thyroid cancer to be an exception. The alterations in precursor cells are likely to occur in infancy or early childhood, and many young children have subclinical cancers (so-called microcarcinomas). Sometimes, these small, indolent thyroid cancers are radiologically or surgically detected in older adults as *incidentalomas*. It became clear that the first (baseline) round of US studies detected thyroid cancers (nearly all PTC) purely due to screening effect. However, the following question arose regarding the future of the children. Would these tiny "cancers" cause morbidity or mortality later in life?

Some of the investigators explained that the first round detected clinically significant microcarcinomas which would continue to grow and cause morbidity in adult life. They expected that the numbers of PTC detected in the next (second) round of screening would sharply decline. The belief that thyroid cancers detected in the first round are at the early stages in the development of aggressive cancers justified surgical treatment and further repeated screening. The need for surgical treatment of these early cancers was conveyed to Fukushima residents by some of the investigators. They did not consider the possibility that US was finding indolent cancers (self-limiting cancers, SLCs) most of which would remain subclinical or slowly progress into symptomatic, but still curable neoplasms. Hence, at this time, overdiagnosis and its harms were not considered. Instead, there was the optimistic belief that early cancer detection was beneficial, and the second round of screening was begun without much discussion.

We now know that the majority of diagnosed PTC become screen-detectable or symptomatic in late adolescence or early adulthood; therefore, one would expect to find increasing numbers of thyroid cancers as Fukushima children enter their teenage years. By analyzing the results of the first round, it would have been easy to predict that the second-round examination would lead to further damage and evoke confusion.[10]

Fig. 4-1 shows the age-specific differences in the number of children with thyroid cancer found in the first-round examination. The number of patients with thyroid cancer increased rapidly in the late teenage years. Calculating the sum of the differences by age, we can predict the number of thyroid cancers detected two years later. The number is 44, which is not small. In fact, fifty-seven children with thyroid cancer were found in the same age group in the second-round examination. This is more than predicted, probably because the interval between the examinations was longer than two years.[11]

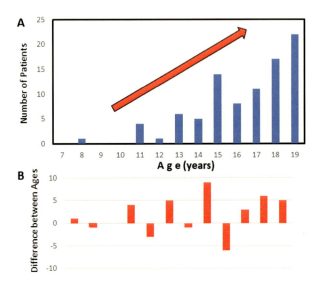

Fig. 4-1 Result of the first-round screening of school children in Fukushima (Adopted from ref.10)

A shows the number of patients diagnosed with thyroid cancer (operated cases), and B shows the subtracted values between each successive age.

The optimistic view that thyroid cancer would rarely be detected in the second-round examination crumbled. At this time, the FHMS leadership acknowledged that, "The increase of thyroid cancer is not due to radiation". However, they seldom attempted to explain the cause of the unexpected increase in thyroid cancer detection. The explanations offered were sometimes confusing or contradictory. The significance of minimal invasion and micrometastasis in subclinical thyroid cancer has not been clarified. Yet, some of the leadership interpreted minimal invasion or micrometastases to mean that the cancer was advanced and in definite need of surgery. At the same time, they stated that small surgical procedures could be done to preserve thyroid function and minimize complications since these cancers were detected at an early stage. In this manner, surgical treatment of small thyroid carcinomas was justified.

Section 5
Prediction of the number of cases detected in the FHMS in the future

From the natural history model based on the fetal cell carcinogenesis theory, Takano predicted the number of patients with thyroid cancer detected in the FHMS. Part of the view is presented in his paper.[9] From the data of autopsy and previous health checkups for college students, about 100 to 200 children and young adults with thyroid cancer are predicted to be found in the first round. Given the rapid growth and relatively high incidence of detectable PTC in the late teens and early adulthood, one predicts that even though the number will somewhat decrease in the second round, the number of detected PTC will still continue to increase each time the examination is repeated. If screening continues for 30 years as planned by the Fukushima Prefecture, as many as 2,000 thyroid cancer patients will be found.

Although decline in participation and, possibly more conservative interpretation of US findings, has led to some decrease in thyroid cancer diagnosis, there has been no data to dispute the assumption that cases of PTC will continue to increase as the thyroid examination continues (Table 2-4). However, there is one piece of data that was unexpected. The average size of thyroid cancer detected in the first round was relatively large at about 1.5 cm.[12] When the cells of these cancers divide three times, they become clinical cancer. For this reason, some experts argued that the patients detected in Fukushima will develop clinical cancer if left untreated. A paper by Miyauchi *et al.*[13] reported evidence to contradict this argument. These investigators found that, not only did most papillary microcarcinomas (PMCs) remain stable into adulthood, but 17% decreased in size during surveillance. We still do not know whether an arbitrary cut off size should be used to distinguish indolent from aggressive cancers, however, a significant number of small thyroid carcinomas will shrink during observation. Therefore, one suspects that many thyroid microcarcinomas remain undetectable or even disappear unless they become discoverable by imaging.

Section 6
Discussion by experts on thyroid cancer overdiagnosis in Fukushima Prefecture

This section describes the discussions of the experts in Fukushima Prefecture. The following discussions have been mainly done in two advisory committees in the FHMS. The Prefectural Oversight Committee for the FHMS (POCF) deals with general matters about the FHMS, and the Task Force for Thyroid Examination (TFTE) deals only with thyroid screening. Details of the discussion were recorded in the minutes of their council meetings.[14, 15]

During the TFTF meeting in 2014, two epidemiologists, Shoichiro Tsugane (National Cancer Institute) and Kenji Shibuya (University of Tokyo), raised some concerns. Their claim was as follows: The design of Fukushima's thyroid examination might not be able to determine the presence or absence of radiation effects, and it is unlikely to improve the participants' health. On the contrary, overdiagnosis could be a disadvantage of the program. Others, mainly surgeons, defended the examination as follows: the harm is negligible because the diagnosis and surgery are done with intense care; if childhood cancers are left untreated, they can transform into anaplastic carcinoma; early diagnosis will improve quality of life (QOL); and the examination will help alleviate the anxiety of Fukushima residents. Some also claimed that continuing data collection should be prioritized over disadvantages to the participants because this data is critical to the mission of clarifying the health effects of radiation exposure.

Shibuya, who recommended reconsidering the thyroid examination, received much criticism, especially from the citizens who complained about nuclear power plants. He had to make excuses for his remarks in his paper.[16] Such fierce criticism has made opponents of the thyroid examination aware of the risks of discussing the problem of overdiagnosis in Fukushima. As a result, these dissidents have become reluctant to discuss this issue.

Table 4-1 Summary of the interim report by the POCF in 2016[17]

1. The increase in thyroid cancer in Fukushima is considered to be a true increase or an increase due to overdiagnosis or screening effect.
2. At present, it is unlikely that the increase is due to radiation exposure.
3. The thyroid examination adds risk to Fukushima residents for "diagnosis and treatment of thyroid cancer that may not have been needed" in addition to "unnecessary radiation exposure."
4. Many Fukushima residents wish to continue the thyroid examination and it is necessary to continue the examination to eliminate their anxiety and to collect data on the effects of the nuclear plant accident.
5. In conclusion, the thyroid examination should be continued after explaining its benefits and harm to the residents.

Following these discussions, the POCF published an interim report on the data from the first-round examination in 2015 (Table 4-1).[17] This report did mention risks of unnecessary treatment but did not delve deeply into an explanation of overdiagnosis. As a result, the thyroid examination proceeded to the third round as planned initially. Based on this report, the Ministry of the Environment and Fukushima Prefecture distributed to related facilities a document stating that starting the thyroid examination in Fukushima was a correct decision, and it should be continued.

In 2017, there was a significant replacement of members of the POCF and TFTE, because a decision was made to include members recommended by related Japanese academic societies. One of the TFTE members, expressed concern that the thyroid examination in Fukushima might have ethical problems. Therefore, the TFTE decided to discuss the ethical issues of the thyroid examination. The discussion was carried out based on the document submitted by Toru Takano and Tomotaka Sobue (Osaka University) (Takano-Sobue recommendations) (Table 4-2).[18, 19]

Table 4-2 Problems designated in Takano-Sobue recommendations

1. Inappropriate informed consent

The harm of ultrasound screening has not been explained to Fukushima residents, and they have been given scientifically incorrect explanations of benefits. Fukushima Prefecture should provide scientifically correct information to the residents.

2. Compulsory school examination

The thyroid examination is currently done at school using school hours. Students and parents have difficulty expressing their intention not to undergo the examination. The examination should be conducted after school or on holidays.

3. Harm of overdiagnosis should be reduced

Possible measures such as using palpation instead of ultrasound, limiting participants by age, or extending intervals between examinations should be considered.

The prefecture refused to discuss the school examination because it worried that the reliability of the obtained data would decrease if any modifications were made to the current examining method. Also, if modifications led to subjects quitting the school examination, the participation rate would decrease. Therefore, only the informed consent was considered for revision.

Table 4-3 Summary of the explanatory document for Fukushima residents

Benefits:
1. When you are worried about the health effects of radiation, and if the examination shows that your thyroid is normal, it may lead to peace of mind and improve your quality of life.
2. Early diagnosis and early treatment reduce the risk of surgical complications, the risk of side effects associated with treatment, and the risk of recurrence.
3. We can obtain information on the health effects of radiation. We can also give such information to people outside the prefecture.

Harm*:
1. Cancers that do not need diagnosis or treatment might be detected.
2. An early cancer diagnosis may result in prolonged treatment and follow-up, increasing psychological burden, and social or economic disadvantages.
3. Nodules and cysts that do not require treatment may be found. As a result, further examinations, such as fine-needle aspiration, may be recommended even for benign diseases. Such a situation may result in psychological and physical burdens for the examinees and their families.

Additional information:
1. In the thyroid US examination, nodules of 5.0 mm or less are not subjected to the secondary examinations. For nodules of 5.1 mm or more, only those suspected of malignancy are subjected to secondary examinations. In this way, measures not to diagnose lesions without the necessity of treatment are taken.
2. Fukushima Prefecture supports medical expenses for treatment and follow-up after the thyroid examination.
3. At Fukushima Medical University, those who undergo secondary examinations are taken care of their anxieties by the professional staff of the mental care support team. In addition, we also offer consultations using a dial to answer medical questions and mental problems related to test results and thyroid diseases. We hold briefing sessions when visiting schools.
4. In the results of the first screening in Fukushima Prefecture, 0.8% of the examinees were recommended secondary examinations, but the remaining 99% or more did not need secondary examinations.
5. In Japan, small surgery is selected for cases other than advanced cancer, and surgery-related complications are less common than in Europe and the United States. Comparing 125 pediatric cases of thyroid cancer operated on at Fukushima Medical University Hospital and cases of thyroid cancer in Belarus after the Chornobyl accident, the outcome of Fukushima Medical University Hospital was far better.
6. Whether it is possible to reduce the mortality rate due to cancer by detecting thyroid cancer with ultrasonography before it becomes symptomatic has not been scientifically clarified.
7. Thyroid cancer generally shows slow progression and low mortality. Cancer is completely cured by treatment unless it is found in advanced stages. The primary treatment is surgery, but observation without surgery may be chosen in the case of small cancers.
8. A cyst is a bag with liquid inside, and it is benign and is often found in healthy people. Since there is only liquid and no cells in a cyst, cancer will not develop from it. A nodule is a change in the density of thyroid cells. A nodule can be benign or malignant, and the majority are benign.

*Fukushima Medical University (FMU) reported an English translation of this document, saying it explains overdiagnosis as harm.[20] However, the actual text does not include the Japanese word corresponding to "overdiagnosis."

After several intense discussions, the prefecture presented a document as a template for the explanation. However, some members expressed fierce dissenting opinions. The principal opinions were that the document contains scientifically incorrect statements to encourage people to undergo the examination, for example, early diagnosis of thyroid cancer reduces recurrence, and it did not refer to the 2018 International Agency for Research on Cancer (IARC) recommendations which stated that thyroid screening is not recommended after a nuclear plant accident.[21] The dissenters also insisted that the document should contain a detailed explanation of the harm of the thyroid examination using the word "overdiagnosis." On the other hand, some members, especially those of the POCF, were concerned that the participation rate would drop if the harm of the examination was overtly posted. No reasonable compromise was reached between the discussants, and finally the Fukushima Prefecture adopted a document that was almost the same as originally proposed (Table 4-3).[22]

After these discussions, the TFTE chairman addressed that medical ethics would no longer be discussed in the TFTE. The ethics committee of FMU approved the research plan. Fukushima Prefecture has since claimed that there is no ethical problem with the thyroid examination because it is conducted with the approval of the ethics committee.

There was no in-depth discussion of the harm of overdiagnosis. There are several reasons for this. First, the members came from various academic societies, and some had a poor understanding of overdiagnosis and medical ethics. This situation made the debate mostly emotional rather than science-based. In addition, the FHMS is a massive organization with a large budget, and various interests exist. It is easy to speculate that some members were expected to give consideration to such interests.

At the POCF meeting in 2024, the results of a questionnaire survey of the subjects and their caregivers of the thyroid examination were reported.[23] The results are shown in Table 4-4. The questionnaire was sent to a total of 16,000 people and the overall response rate was 22%. These results highlighted the ethical problems with the thyroid examination in Fukushima.

Following the POCF's guidance, Fukushima Prefecture and FMU are distributing pamphlets on the thyroid examination to the residents (Table 4-3). They explain the benefits of having a thyroid examination, such as peace of mind, early diagnosis, and understanding the effects of radiation exposure, however, all of these are considered to be scientifically incorrect and inappropriate. Looking at the results of the survey, caregivers, in particular, understand these explanations very well and, as a result, believe that it is a good thing to have their children undergo thyroid screening. It is also noteworthy that many people said they want to take the examination because it is done at school. Thus, it is evident that school checkups are a factor in the spread of damage.

Table 4-4 Results of the questionnaire survey of the residents[23]

		Caregiver		Subject	
Age of the subject		-15	16-17	16-17	18-
Response rate		30.2%	27.9%	22.3%	11.0%
Recognize the benefits and harm of the thyroid examination		55.1%	58.1%	34.7%	38.1%
Want to be examined in the future		70.2%	61.8%	59.4%	43.5%
Reason	Feel safe after the examination	84.2%	84.5%	71.8%	67.7%
	Early diagnosis is possible	63.9%	63.7%	42.2%	52.6%
	Possible to know the effect of radiation exposure	50.8%	54.9%	39.3%	35.4%
	Being examined at school	47.6%	39.6%	42.3%	-
Don't want to be examined in the future		1.6%	2.2%	14.3%	27.0%
Reason	Risk of overdiagnosis	26.3%	20.8%	3.1%	8.4%

Although a minimal number of caregivers do not want their children to undergo the examination, a certain percentage of them cite overdiagnosis as the reason. Fukushima Prefecture has avoided explaining the overdiagnosis in detail to the residents. Therefore, it is assumed that these people are obtaining information on the thyroid examination from sources other than those provided by Fukushima Prefecture.

The general public's understanding of overdiagnosis is very poor, and the situation was such that when a committee member brought up the issue of overdiagnosis, that person would be accused of concealing damage caused by the nuclear accident. In fact, at meetings with media reporters, committee members who mentioned overdiagnosis were not only repeatedly denounced but were even asked to resign. Under these circumstances, some committee members, who understood the harms of overdiagnosis, were reluctant to voice their opinions.

Section 7
The damages of overdiagnosis are now spreading outside the FHMS

The number of children diagnosed with thyroid cancer in the third round of the thyroid examination has plummeted.[24] However, this might not mean that the damage caused by overdiagnosis has subsided. In the thyroid examination in Fukushima, thyroid US is first performed as a screening test (primary examination), and only children with abnormalities undergo another thyroid US (confirmatory examination). The children who are determined to need a definitive diagnosis by this examination will undergo fine-needle aspiration cytology (FNAC) (see Chapter 2). In the third-round examination, a decrease in the participation rates of the confirmatory examination and FNAC was evident. As a result, the number of children suspected to have thyroid cancer decreased considerably (Table 4-5).

Table 4-5 Participation rate of the thyroid examination in Fukushima

		1st round	2nd round	3rd round
Primary Examination	Subjects	367637	381244	336667
	Participants	300472 (81.7%)	270552 (71.0%)	217922 (64.7%)
Confirmatory Examination	Subjects	2293	2230	1502
	Participants	2130 (92.9%)	1877 (84.2%)	1104 (73.5%)
	FNAC	547 (25.7%)	207 (11.0%)	79 (7.2%)
Number of the children suspected to have thyroid cancer		116	71	31

It is essential to clarify the reason for decline in participation. The children in Fukushima have already experienced the thyroid examination many times. What happens to a child when an abnormality is repeatedly found by US and follow-up is recommended, but the parents have not been informed of the risk of overdiagnosis? The family might want more information about the diagnosis and therapy. Fukushima is mainly a rural area with relatively few hospitals. Tokyo is one and half-hour's distance by Shinkansen train from Fukushima, and Tokyo has many hospitals and thyroid specialists. Likely, the parents of children with abnormalities detected during the primary examination of the third round would seek specialty consultations and definitive diagnoses in Tokyo rather than undergo follow-up US in Fukushima. It has been confirmed that there are at least 20 children with thyroid cancer found outside of the tabulation of the count of the FHMS.

A survey by Sobue Tomotaka *et al.* (Osaka University) found that the number of thyroid US examinations claims in medical insurance records has tripled in the

Fukushima Prefecture and doubled in neighboring prefectures after the Great East Japan Earthquake (personal communication). These findings suggest that the damage caused by thyroid cancer overdiagnosis is no longer within the framework of the FHMS. Even if the thyroid examination in the FHMS is discontinued, overdiagnosis will continue owing to families seeking evaluation for thyroid cancer outside of the FHMS.

One of the reasons for the increase in the number of thyroid US examinations conducted in Fukushima Prefecture is the subsidy project of Fukushima Prefecture. Fukushima Prefecture and the Fukushima Medical Association are conducting two subsidy projects to meet the increasing demand for thyroid US in the prefecture. One is a subsidy for purchasing thyroid US equipment, and the other is for a course to train medical professionals to perform thyroid US. These subsidies have made it possible for thyroid US to be performed in many hospitals in Fukushima. Given the availability of US machines and training, doctors are likely to perform thyroid US more frequently in order to both meet patients' demands and increase profits. Overuse of US leads to overdiagnosis and overtreatment of thyroid nodules as occurred in South Korea (see Chapter 1). Such a movement also proves that Fukushima Prefecture and related experts do not understand the nature of overdiagnosis correctly.

Consequences of the thyroid examination in Fukushima have spread throughout Japan. The launch of the FHMS in Fukushima Prefecture has led to a widespread misconception that children and adolescents should undergo thyroid US screening for early detection of thyroid cancer after a nuclear accident. As a result, thyroid US screening is also being conducted on children and adolescents outside Fukushima Prefecture. Some screenings are planned by local governments outside Fukushima Prefecture as health checkups for the residents, for example, in Marumori Town, Miyagi Prefecture, and Kitaibaraki City, Ibaraki Prefecture.[25, 26] Many health checkups with thyroid US are financed by soliciting donations from anti-nuclear citizen groups. These examinations have already been performed on tens of thousands of people, and unfortunately, many children and adolescents with thyroid cancer have been found.

References
1. Tokonami S, *et al.* Thyroid doses for evacuees from the Fukushima nuclear accident. *Sci Rep* 2:507, 2012.
2. Nagataki S, Yamashita S. Thirty years after the Chernobyl Nuclear Power Plant Accident: Contribution from Japan—"Confirming the increase of childhood thyroid cancer." In: Thyroid cancer and nuclear accidents: Long-term aftereffects of

Chernobyl and Fukushima (1st ed.). Academic Press, pp.11-20, 2017.
3. Shiraishi H. Review of the examination method behind the scenes of 250 children with thyroid cancer. *Sekai* 942:238-45, 2021(in Japanese).
4. Kondo T, *et al*. Pathogenetic mechanisms in thyroid follicular-cell neoplasia. *Nat Rev Cancer* 6:292-306, 2006.
5. Suzuki S. Childhood and adolescent thyroid cancer in Fukushima after the Fukushima Daiichi Nuclear Power Plant accident: 5 years on. *Clin Oncol* 28:263-71, 2016.
6. Tsuda T, *et al*. Thyroid cancer detection by ultrasound among residents ages 18 years and younger in Fukushima, Japan: 2011 to 2014. *Epidemiology* 27:316-22, 2016.
7. Cléro E, *et al*. Lessons learned from Chernobyl and Fukushima on thyroid cancer screening and recommendations in case of a future nuclear accident. *Environ Int*. 146:106230, 2021.
8. Welch HG, Black WC. Overdiagnosis in cancer. *J Natl Cancer Inst* 102:605-13, 2010.
9. Takano T. Natural history of thyroid cancer. *Endocr J* 64:237-44, 2017.
10. Takano T. Overdiagnosis of juvenile thyroid cancer. *Eur Thyroid J* 9:124-31, 2020.
11. Ohtsuru A, *et al*. Incidence of thyroid cancer among children and young adults in Fukushima, Japan, screened with 2 rounds of ultrasonography within 5 years of the 2011 Fukushima Daiichi nuclear power station accident. *JAMA Otolaryngol Head Neck Surg*145:4-11, 2019.
12. Suzuki S, *et al*. Histopathological analysis of papillary thyroid carcinoma detected during ultrasound screening examinations in Fukushima. *Cancer Sci* 110:817-27, 2019.
13. Miyauchi A, *et al*. Natural history of papillary thyroid microcarcinoma: kinetic analysis on tumor volume during active surveillance and before presentation. *Surg*ery 165:25-30, 2019.
14. Fukushima Prefecture. Fukushima, Japan: The Prefectural Oversight Committee for the FHMS (in Japanese). [internet, cited 2024 July 15] Available from: https://www.pref.fukushima.lg.jp/site/portal/kenkocyosa-kentoiinkai.html.
15. Fukushima Prefecture. Fukushima, Japan: The Task Force for Thyroid Examination (in Japanese). [internet, cited 2024 July 15] Available from: https://www.pref.fukushima.lg.jp/sec/21045b/kenkocyosa-kentoiinkai-b.html.
16. Shibuya K, *et al*. Time to reconsider thyroid screening in Fukushima. *Lancet* 383: 1883-4, 2014.
17. Fukushima Prefecture. Fukushima, Japan: Interim report of the Fukushima Health

Management Survey (in Japanese). [internet, cited 2024 July 15] Available from: https://www.pref.fukushima.lg.jp/uploaded/attachment/158522.pdf.
18. Fukushima Prefecture. Fukushima, Japan: Ethical issues and improvement proposals for the thyroid ultrasound examination in the Fukushima Health Management Survey (in Japanese). [internet, cited 2024 July 15] Available from: https://www.pref.fukushima.lg.jp/uploaded/attachment/278764.pdf.
19. Fukushima Prefecture. Fukushima, Japan: Problems and improvement proposals for the implementation system and method of the thyroid ultrasound examination in the Fukushima Health Management Survey (in Japanese). [internet, cited 2024 July 15] Available from: https://www.pref.fukushima.lg.jp/uploaded/attachment/295104.pdf.
20. Shimura H, *et al*. A comprehensive review of the progress and evaluation of the thyroid ultrasound examination program, the Fukushima Health Management Survey. *J Epidemiol* 32 (Suppl.XII):S23-35, 2022.
21. Togawa K, *et al*. Long-term strategies for thyroid health monitoring after nuclear accidents: recommendations from an Expert Group convened by IARC. *Lancet Oncol* 19:1280-3, 2018.
22. Fukushima Prefecture. Fukushima, Japan: Fukushima Heath Management Suvey: Thyroid examination. Benefits and harms of the examination (in Japanese). [internet, cited 2024 July 15] Available from: https://fukushima-mimamori.jp/thyroid-examination/uploads/merit_demerit_booklet_01.pdf.
23. Fukushima Prefecture. Fukushima, Japan: Results of the questionnaire survey regarding the thyroid examination (in Japanese). [internet, cited 2024 July 15] Available from: https://www.pref.fukushima.lg.jp/uploaded/attachment/611554.pdf.
24. Fukushima Prefecture. Fukushima, Japan: Materials from the 42nd meeting of the Prefectural Oversight Committee for the FHMS (in Japanese). [internet, cited 2024 July 15] Available from: https://www.pref.fukushima.lg.jp/sec/21045b/kenkocyosa-kentoiinkai-42.html.
25. Marumori Town. Miyagi, Japan: Marumori Town Thyroid Examination Guidelines (in Japanese). [internet, cited 2024 July 15] Available from: http://www.town.marumori.miyagi.jp/reiki/reiki_honbun/c218RG00000366.html.
26. Kitaibaraki City. Ibaraki, Japan: Result of thyroid US examination in Kitaibaraki City (in Japanese). [internet, cited 2024 July 15] Available from: https://www.city.kitaibaraki.lg.jp/docs/2021011200010/file_contents/2526.pdf.

Chapter 5
Disagreements among academicians regarding the thyroid ultrasound examination and overdiagnosis

As of early 2024, over 300 cases of thyroid cancer have been detected as a result of the thyroid examination in the Fukushima Health Management Survey (FHMS). Additional cases are being diagnosed outside the FHMS (see Chapter 6). It has become clear to some physicians involved in the screening program that the thyroid examination has resulted in overdiagnosis and psychosocial harm. Yet, many Japanese academic experts oppose the view that overdiagnosis has occurred, and the methodology of the program remains unchanged. This chapter discusses the views of members of Japanese academic societies and scientific organizations in regard to the thyroid examination and reviews the arguments in favor of continuing the program. Also, the opposing arguments by some experts, especially the members of the Japanese Consortium for Juvenile Thyroid Cancer (JCJTC) are given. The chapter also explains how Japanese preventing overdiagnosis movements are trying to work to educate the public and effect modifications to the thyroid examination program. The statements and recommendations of some international expert groups are also reviewed.

Section 1
Recommendations by international organizations

Experts/researchers on both sides of any argument must address both self-interest and personal biases. Similarly, the mission of the editorial staff of scientific journals should be to publish well-written, cogent manuscripts from both sides of controversies regardless of personal biases or interests of associated medical societies. The hoped-for outcome is to generate discussion by neutral expert groups and collaboration between opposing sides to maximize benefits and minimize harm to patients. Both sides should avoid cherry-picking references or portions of reports in order to, as Hofmann puts it, *"facting interests"* instead of reporting *"interesting facts"*.[1]

Recommendations made by both the US Preventive Service Task Force (USPSTF) on screening for thyroid cancer and the International Agency for Cancer Research (IARC) Expert Group on Thyroid Health Monitoring after Nuclear Accidents have often been used to further arguments by both the FHMS and those concerned about overdiagnosis. Before presenting claims made by Japanese experts, it is important to review what was said by both of these organizations in order to understand how statements by the same organizations can be used to support two sides of the FHMS's thyroid examination controversy.[2-4]

The USPSTF recommends against screening for thyroid cancer in asymptomatic adults because it concluded, based on indirect evidence, that the potential harms are at least moderate and the benefits small, at best. Harms include overdiagnosis and unnecessary treatment (overtreatment). Costs were not considered. Population (mass) screening of asymptomatic children is not addressed in the USPSTF. The USPSTF does state that their recommendations do not apply to people with a history of childhood radiation, exposure to radioactive fallout, or a history of familial or genetic disorders that increase the risk of thyroid cancer. At the same time, the USPSTF states that they did not find studies that compared surgery to surveillance and admits that there is still a need for studies to establish whether screening people with a history of exposure to radiation is beneficial.[2] Systematic review by the USPSTF found no studies comparing outcomes of thyroid screening versus unscreened, and no studies directly examined the harms of overdiagnosis or screening in general.[3] The USPSTF reports indicate a significant lack of knowledge regarding the outcome benefits of thyroid ultrasound (US) screening and acknowledge the potential for overdiagnosis and overtreatment.

The IARC Expert Group on Thyroid Health Monitoring after Nuclear Accidents is a collaboration of international scientists with expertise in a variety of different fields.

These experts were assembled to deal with the problem of thyroid health evaluation after nuclear accidents.[4] IARC recommends against population (mass) screening for thyroid cancer after a nuclear accident because the harms are deemed to outweigh the benefits. Screening is defined as the recruitment of all people living in a defined area for palpation or US evaluation followed by other testing. Screening eligibility is defined by region not by other factors such as radiation dose assessment. IARC acknowledges that screening children and adolescents without regard to dose exposure has the potential to result in overdiagnosis without any health benefits.

It is still unknown whether there is any benefit to US screening of asymptomatic children, adolescents, or young adults exposed to higher levels of radiation at a young age. There is no evidence that radiation-associated thyroid cancer is more aggressive than spontaneous thyroid cancer. Both share excellent long-term prognoses. IARC does acknowledge that consideration can be given to long-term monitoring of people considered high-risk. It states that children exposed to radiation doses of 100-500mGy or more are considered at high risk for thyroid cancer.

Monitoring is not the same as screening. First and foremost, monitoring is a purely elective procedure. Educational programs including health literacy and discussion of harms and benefits are prerequisites for participation, and participation should be completely voluntary. Subjects are recruited based on estimated dose exposure and risk rather than population in general. There should be registration of participation and central data collection.

IARC acknowledges that there are significant gaps in knowledge. At the current time, there is no way to assess whether a thyroid cancer diagnosed via US and fine-needle aspiration cytology (FNAC) will or will not progress. There is evidence that nearly all papillary microcarcinoma (PMC) are either non-progressive or indolent, and the prognosis is excellent even in the presence of metastases, especially in children.[5, 6] The risk of harms of overdiagnosis and overtreatment exist, and subjects participating in monitoring should be aware of the risks and the possibility of no benefit other than the acquisition of data for research.

It should also be noted that IARC experts are careful to state that their recommendations are not directed against current ongoing studies (such as the thyroid examination in Fukushima) and that the report is not an evaluation of thyroid health monitoring activities that were implemented after the past nuclear accidents. IARC also states that final decisions regarding monitoring should lie with the respective governments, relevant authorities, and the affected societies. However, IARC experts also state that the guiding principle of any health-related intervention should be to "maximize benefit and minimize harm."[4]

Although IARC does not direct its recommendations to ongoing projects and acknowledges the right of the government, local experts, and affected inhabitants to make policy decisions, IARC experts clearly state that the harms of population screening likely outweigh the benefits. Thus, these statements should not be interpreted as a green light for continuing the thyroid examination in the FHMS unmodified but should be interpreted as justification for the government and related experts to re-evaluate the examination, discuss the observed harms, investigate whether there has been evidence of benefits, improve thyroid health literacy among participants including the concept of overdiagnosis, and ensure that continued participation is truly voluntary without stigmatization for non-participation.

Section 2
The Japanese academic societies' viewpoints

In the Japanese academic societies, there has been little discussion about the problem of overdiagnosis of thyroid cancer in Fukushima. In 2017, Sanae Midorikawa and Akira Ohtsuru, who were in charge of the thyroid examination at Fukushima Medical University (FMU), first mentioned concerns about thyroid cancer overdiagnosis in Fukushima during a symposium at the annual meeting of the Japan Endocrine Society. Their remarks attracted the attention of the general public as well as academicians, and their remarks were criticized by some citizen groups who accused them of attempting to discontinue the thyroid examination in Fukushima. Since then, FMU has requested its members to avoid further discussion of overdiagnosis at academic conferences.

In Japanese medical societies and their associated journals, thyroid experts have repeatedly defended the US examination and surgical treatment of thyroid cancers. They insist that overdiagnosis is not occurring.[7] Subsequently, there has been little criticism of the thyroid examination or mention of overdiagnosis. Table 5-1 summarizes the experts' views.

Table 5-1 Japanese experts' views in support of the thyroid examination in Fukushima[7-9]

1. Pathological findings after surgery show metastasis and invasion in many cases, so it is judged that there is no overdiagnosed case.
2. Unlike other countries diagnosis and surgery are performed sophisticatedly in Japan according to Japanese guidelines, so the harm of overdiagnosis is negligible.
3. All small childhood thyroid cancers found in Fukushima are future clinical cases that were found at a very early stage.
4. By finding thyroid cancer at an early stage, small surgery can be performed, and as a result, surgical complications, hypothyroidism, and recurrence can be prevented.
5. The definition of overdiagnosis does not apply to the thyroid US examination which is aimed at reducing residents' anxiety.

Section 3
Statement from the Science Council of Japan

The Science Council of Japan (SCJ) is the representative organization of Japanese scientists, and includes experts from all fields of the sciences, national and international. The SCJ is under the jurisdiction of the Prime Minister but operates independently of the government. It functions to deliberate on important issues using science to solve problems and offer policy recommendations to the government and the public. The SCJ has issued several reports about thyroid cancer in Fukushima. The final report of 2017 made a very preliminary decision on the overdiagnosis problem.[10] While expressing concern about the disadvantages of overdiagnosis, the report only mentioned that further discussion should be carried out in the future and did not point out any specific problems with Fukushima's thyroid examination or propose improvement plans.

Section 4
Biased tone in Japanese academic journals

Some authors concerned about the harms of the thyroid examination in Fukushima have experienced difficulty publishing such concerns in Japanese academic journals.

Toru Takano (Rinku General Medical Center) submitted a paper to Endocrine Journal, the official English-language journal of the Japan Endocrine Society. The manuscript addresses the potential for overdiagnosis and stigmatization caused by the thyroid examination in Fukushima, stresses the need for discussion of overdiagnosis, and reminds that the first priority of the FHMS is to protect children's health and welfare. It was rejected after being reviewed by a single Japanese reviewer. A reason for rejection was given as a lack of a correct understanding of the FHMS. This paper was ultimately published in a European journal without any major modifications. [11]

In 2021, a report of the cytologic examinations performed in the FHMS was published in Endocrine Journal.[12] Most of the authors were engaged in the FHMS at the time. Although the focus of the article is to report fine-needle aspiration cytology (FNAC) findings using the Bethesda System, the publication contains some statements giving support to the FHMS. Several authors submitted letters disagreeing with statements in this paper. All but one were rejected after being reviewed by Japanese reviewers. The reason for rejection was a lack of correct understanding of the FHMS or because their arguments were not suitable to discuss in Endocrine Journal. The published dissenting letter discusses what the authors believe to be flaws in the article's statements in support of continuing the thyroid examination.[13] The arguments in the original paper and the letter's counterarguments are summarized below.

1. **Although the USPSTF recommends against screening for thyroid cancer in asymptomatic adults, this statement does not apply to those at high risk owing to the history of exposure to ionizing radiation.**
   The article fails to acknowledge that absorbed and effective radiation levels in Fukushima have been estimated to be very low and not at levels that would place residents at high risk for thyroid cancer.

2. **Overtreatment does not occur in the survey because the majority of patients who undergo surgery are treated with lobectomy.**
   Smaller surgical procedures (hemithyroidectomy) should still be considered overtreatment if the resected lesion is self-limiting or indolent.

3. **The survey results will contribute to future research on childhood and adolescent thyroid cancer.**
   If a study is performed solely for research purposes, participation must be voluntary, and subjects should be aware that the study is intended for

research. There may be no benefits, and there is the potential for harm including overdiagnosis.

It is ultimately up to the editor-in-chief to decide whether or not to accept a submitted paper. However, regarding issues with discrepant opinions among experts, such as the thyroid examination in Fukushima, academic journals should include arguments from both sides and encourage collaboration to maximize benefits, minimize harms and allow for informed and shared decision-making. From this point of view, it was not desirable to dismiss most of the counterarguments to the thyroid examination in Fukushima. Furthermore, instead of unilaterally rejecting adoption based on the opinion of a single domestic reviewer, overseas reviewers should have been invited to provide a multifaceted approach.

Unfortunately, Japanese academic journals have not been actively discussing the harmful effects of the FHMS so far, and information tends to be biased toward supporting the continuation of the thyroid examination.

Section 5
Conflicts in Japanese thyroid-related academic societies

The Japan Thyroid Association (JTA) has been heavily involved in initiating and continuing the FHMS. Although some members had requested a public discussion on the issue of Fukushima's thyroid examination, the Board of Directors has not admitted to starting an argument. Thus little discussion followed.

The JTA certifies thyroid specialists, and an annual examination is conducted on eligible individuals. The designated learning material is the Guidebook for Thyroid Specialists, which is edited by the JTA members.[14] The JTA has instructed the question creators to ask questions for the specialist examination based on the content contained in this book. In the revised second edition of this book which was published in 2018, the FHMS was newly adopted as an item that specialists should know, and a chapter was devoted to explaining it. It states that the increase in the number of thyroid cancers detected in the thyroid examination in the FHMS is due to a screening or harvesting effect and that overdiagnosis and overtreatment are not occurring. It lists five reasons for this, as listed below.
1) Borderline lesions such as noninvasive follicular thyroid neoplasm with papillary-like nuclear features (NIFTP) were not included in the operated cases.

2) Diagnostic procedures strictly follow the guidelines to prevent overdiagnosis.
3) Unlike precedents in countries such as South Korea, small thyroid cancers are not diagnosed in Fukushima.
4) All resected cancers smaller than 10 mm had metastasis or invasion.
5) Total thyroidectomy is avoided whenever possible.

These views remained unchanged even after the opinions of the international expert teams, such as IARC, the United Nations Scientific Committee on the Effects of Atomic Radiation (UNSCEAR), and Nuclear Emergency Situation-Improvement of Medical and Health Surveillance (SHAMISEN), were issued. As a result of such scientifically incorrect education being provided to academic members, many Japanese thyroid experts either have avoided pointing out mistakes and feigned indifference to the problem in Fukushima or have a mistaken understanding.

Triggered by requests from general members in 2020, the editorial board of the Journal of the Japan Thyroid Association, which belongs to the JTA, published a special topic devoted to the discussion of the overdiagnosis of thyroid cancer. Sanae Midorikawa, who moved to Miyagi Gakuin Women's University from FMU, became the editor-in-charge. The topic was published in April 2021. In this special topic, not only thyroid experts but experts in epidemiology, radiation, and medical ethics, including an overseas expert, Wendy A. Rogers (Macquarie University, Australia), contributed. Some clearly expressed concerns about the thyroid examination in Fukushima.[15-19]

Immediately after its publication, the Board of Directors of the JTA announced that the contents of this special feature are the opinions of only a limited number of the JTA members. Furthermore, it said that the JTA had always given special consideration to the overdiagnosis problem and would continue to support the FHMS.[20] The Board of Directors also announced that under its initiative without the involvement of the editorial board, another special topic would be published in the JTA journal in which articles would convey an accurate portrayal of Fukushima's thyroid examination. In October of the same year, this special topic was published. Some papers claim that Fukushima's thyroid examination does not cause any problematic overdiagnosis because it strictly follows the Japanese guidelines, and the pathological findings proved that none of the cases that underwent surgery were likely to have been overdiagnosed.[8, 9] Akira Ohtsuru, who moved to Nagasaki University from FMU, submitted letters that were against the views described above. They were accepted for publication, and in April 2022, his letters were published with counterarguments by the authors of the special feature.[21-24]

As mentioned above, at the JTA, there was a sharp conflict between the board members trying to assist the FHMS and some general members concerned about overdiagnosis. Most members of the JTA are trying to avoid scientific debate to avoid getting drawn into the conflict between the two sides. Therefore, there has been no criticism of the Fukushima thyroid examination at the JTA meetings.

An organization called *Save the Children from Overdiagnosis* (SCO) was formed to convey scientifically accurate information about the thyroid examination and overdiagnosis. This organization was established mainly by the JTA members and operates anonymously. SCO utilizes social media such as YouTube, Instagram, and X to disseminate information. It has released animations that briefly explain overdiagnosis in a way that the general public can understand.[25] It also introduces experts' views on the thyroid examination in Fukushima and learning materials on social media. [26, 27]

Not only JTA but other academic societies have been reluctant to convey information on the damage caused by the overdiagnosis or overtreatment of thyroid cancer in Fukushima. Rather, some academic societies have increased technical guidance on thyroid US and FNAC to meet the growing demand for thyroid US. The Japanese Association of Breast and Thyroid Sonology (JABTS) established a novel specialist training program for FNAC in 2020.[28] This program is one of the reasons for an increase in the number of unnecessary thyroid US examinations in Fukushima and neighboring prefectures.

There are two theoretical reasons for this reluctance. First, some academics have significant stakes in the success of the FHMS because they were involved in its initial planning. Second, thyroid US is a valuable source of income for hospitals; therefore, disseminating information on harms may be undesirable. Academic societies should act based on scientific facts. However, since there are various conflicts of interest, it seems that priority has been given to not changing the original policy without discussing the problems to avoid erupting disputes.

Section 6
Establishment of the Japan Consortium of Juvenile Thyroid Cancer

In 2020, some experts who felt a sense of crisis in the situation in Japan formed a new academic society named the Japan Consortium of Juvenile Thyroid Cancer (JCJTC).[29] The JCJTC is composed of experts from various fields in Japan who have no conflict of interest regarding the overdiagnosis problem in Fukushima. Some overseas experts were also invited to participate. The JCJTC aims to disseminate accurate scientific information through social media, hold international symposiums, and create recommendations for optimizing domestic medical care.

The home page of JCJTC is a valuable source for overseas experts to find out about the status of the overdiagnosis of thyroid cancer in Fukushima. A Japanese version of the video of the international symposium is also available, helping the general public to understand overdiagnosis. For example, Sanae Midorikawa (Miyagi Gakuin Women's University) has presented roundtable discussions with Fukushima mothers, Toru Takano (Rinku General Medical Center) has chaired similar discussions with Japanese medical students, and a Japanese nursing student who participated in the Fukushima thyroid examination has related her experiences and recent activities.[30-34]

Section 7
Reports from international organizations

Although the Japanese academic community has taken almost no action on overdiagnosis, various international organizations have published reports on thyroid cancer in Fukushima, which are partly described in Section 1. In 2017, SHAMISEN presented recommendations on how to respond after a nuclear accident. These recommendations were published as a paper in 2020 as part of a SHAMISEN special issue.[35] SHAMISEN recommendations are very similar to those later issued by IARC experts. Based on the Fukushima screening experience, the SHAMISEN consortium advises against population thyroid cancer screening because the physical and psychological harms are likely to be greater than the benefits. The group stresses the ethical principle that post-nuclear accident activities must do "more good than harm." Psychological and socioeconomic issues must be considered, and activities must preserve the dignity and autonomy of the affected population.

In 2017, with the support of the Ministry of the Environment of Japan, IARC established an international expert group, Thyroid Health Monitoring after Nuclear Accidents (TM-NUC), which studies the ideal way of thyroid monitoring after a nuclear accident. In 2018, TM-NUC issued recommendations on how to respond after a nuclear accident.[4,36] Some of their recommendations have been discussed in Section 1 as well as the difference between screening and monitoring. At the request of the Ministry of the Environment of Japan, the IARC TM-NUC recommendations were added with a sentence stating that they do not apply to projects that are already underway. A summary of the recommendations is shown in Table 5-2. Similar to SHAMISEN's recommendations and as discussed previously, IARC TM-NUC recommends against population screening after a nuclear accident but states that monitoring could be considered. [4, 36] Both SHAMISEN and IARC TM-NUC statements encourage discussion and potential changes to the thyroid examination. Not only must there be efforts to ensure that the harms do not outweigh the benefits, but as stated by SHAMISEN, there must be an educational program, and the autonomy and dignity of the affected population must be preserved. [37] Thus, participation in the thyroid examination should be entirely voluntary with respect to decisions not to participate, and all subjects must be educated in thyroid health and informed of the risks and benefits.

In 2013, prior to the SHAMSEN and IARC publications, UNSCEAR reported that the thyroid cancer found in Fukushima is unlikely to be due to radiation exposure. UNSCEAR issued an updated report (report 2020/2021). UNSCLEAR's opinion that radiation levels were too low to cause thyroid cancer remains unchanged, and in the updated report, UNSCEAR states that the thyroid cancer found in Fukushima might be overdiagnosed owing to US screening.[38]

UNSCEAR Outreach Event in Japan 2022 was held in July 2022. The principal members who prepared the UNSCEAR report held a press conference in Tokyo and attended town meetings in Fukushima and Iwaki. However, this event was rarely reported in the national media. Exceptionally, the Tokyo Shimbun covered the event extensively, but it was critical of UNSCEAR. In the article, some citizen groups and Japanese researchers point out some mistakes in UNSCEAR's report, and the representative of a citizen group said that the content of the report promotes discrimination and prejudice against Fukushima residents. The article also states that one of the patients diagnosed with thyroid cancer in Fukushima said it is hard for her to accept the conclusion that her thyroid cancer is unrelated to exposure because it seems that such a conclusion was drawn without sufficient scientific data. Later, the Asahi Shimbun, one of Japan's main stream journal, also ran an article about the UNSCEAR report. It introduces an epidemiologist's view that the UNSCEAR report is scientifically flawed and that the occurrence of overdiagnosis is not likely.

The chairman of the Task Force for Thyroid Examination (TFTE), commented on the UNSCEAR report. He partly disagreed with UNSCEAR's conclusion, saying that without long-term observation, it is impossible to know if overdiagnosis is actually occurring. He argued that the investigation in Fukushima should continue for at least 20 years to clarify the matter. The chairman of the Prefectural Oversight Committee for the FHMS (POCF), said that POCF's view is not necessarily the same as UNSCEAR's. He also stated that the FHMS's primary mission is to respond to Fukushima residents' concerns and protect their health.

Section 8
Discussions on the IARC's recommendations

The details of the IARC definitions and recommendations have been described in Section 1. SHAMISEN and UNSCEAR reports have also been addressed previously. These international reports, especially the IARC report, were welcomed by some domestic experts who consider overdiagnosis a severe problem. However, as mentioned previously, some experts made selective use of and misinterpretation of IARC comments to support the thyroid examination in Fukushima.

In 2021, the third International Symposium on the FHMS was held in Fukushima, and those who engaged in the FHMS and chief members of the related Japanese academic societies participated.[39] In this symposium, the IARC recommendations were introduced to the audience; however, the contents were different from the original ones.

The exposure doses of children in Fukushima were much lower than those in Chornobyl (<<100 mGy); thus, IARC does not consider these children at high risk for thyroid cancer. Two mistakes in the presentation of the IARC recommendations are illustrated in Table 5-2. First, IARC recommends against population (mass) screening after a nuclear accident under any conditions. IARC does suggest that *voluntary* participation in thyroid monitoring could be offered to those exposed to doses ≥100-500 mGy. The symposium experts explained that IARC would recommend conducting monitoring in Fukushima. During the symposium, no one pointed out the mistakes, and the discussions continued. Also, there was confusion about the terms monitoring versus screening. During the symposium, the experts explained that the thyroid examination in Fukushima is monitoring but not screening according to the IARC definitions.

In 2022, the annual meeting of the Japan Pediatric Society, sponsored by FMU, was held in Fukushima, and a symposium on the thyroid examination in Fukushima was set up. In this symposium, the same modified recommendations were presented again. Further, one of the Japanese speakers explained that the IARC report clearly states that the IARC recommendations are not views on ongoing projects like those in Fukushima and emphasized that the thyroid examination in Fukushima should be decided independently of the IARC recommendations.

Some experts made similar claims at POCF or TFTE. They stated that the IARC report was prepared without considering the situation in Fukushima and stated that its recommendations have nothing to do with the thyroid examination in Fukushima, so Fukushima residents do not need to know their content.

Table 5-2 Comparison of the original IARC recommendations and the recommendations presented at academic meetings in Japan

IARC recommendations
1. The Expert Group **recommends against** population thyroid **screening** after a nuclear accident.
2. The Expert Group recommends that consideration be given to offering a long-term thyroid **monitoring** (those exposed in utero or during childhood or adolescence with a thyroid dose of **100–500 mGy or more**).

Recommendations presented in academic meetings in Japan
1. No population-based thyroid **screening** after a nuclear accident where thyroid doses are below **100–500 mSv**.
2. Consideration should be given to offering a long-term thyroid **monitoring** program for higher-risk individuals after a nuclear accident.

Section 9
Discussions on active surveillance and the use of the term "overdiagnosis"

Active surveillance (AS) of PMC was first attempted and established in Japan and is considered one of the most outstanding achievements by Japanese thyroid experts. As a result, when some became concerned about the harm caused by overdiagnosis in the FHMS, there was a prevailing opinion that there would be no problem if AS is appropriately implemented.

However, AS has been applied only to adults. The ideal candidate is considered to be an older adult without evidence of metastases, and there is, as yet, little or no data on AS in children. Furthermore, in the case of children, AS has the potential for major harm. The observation period for children will be exceptionally long. This can adversely affect the quality of life (QOL) for young people seeking education, social interaction and, eventually, marriage. Additionally, it can cause financial disadvantages such as difficulty obtaining insurance or loans. Some experts have pointed out these problems, but many others, especially surgeons, claim that such adverse effects are negligible. Such discussions are recorded in the minutes of the POCF and TFTE meetings.[40, 41]

Also, there is confusion concerning the definition of overdiagnosis. Formerly, overdiagnosis was used synonymously with misdiagnosis or misclassification. Overdiagnosis is now defined as "labeling of a person with a disease or abnormal condition that would not have caused the person harm if left undiscovered" (see Chapter 1). In 2022, the Japan Association of Endocrine Surgeons and the Japanese Society of Thyroid Surgery published a special topic on the FHMS in their official journal. Some papers were written by the experts involved in the FHMS. They claimed that the term overdiagnosis is misused in Japan, and it should be used only in the sense of pathological misdiagnosis but not in the manner defined by Medical Subjects Headings (MeSH), as those who criticize the FHMS use it.[42] Furthermore, the preface of this special topic states that the criticism that the FHMS is causing overdiagnosis is very annoying.

Although thyroid health education, including the concept of overdiagnosis, is a necessary prerequisite for informed consent and shared decision making, the fact that the experts supporting the FHMS in Japan have changed the definition of overdiagnosis to suit their purposes has been a significant obstacle to education of the general public.

References

1. Hofmann B. Fake facts and alternate truths in medical research. **BMC Medical Ethics** 19:4-9, 2018.
2. US Preventive Services Task Force. Screening for thyroid cancer: US Preventive Services Task Force recommendation statement. **JAMA** 317:1882-7, 2017.
3. Lin JS, *et al.* Screening for thyroid cancer updated evidence report and systematic review for the US Preventive Services Task Force. **JAMA** 3017:1888-1903, 2017.
4. International Agency for Research on Cancer. Lyon, France: Thyroid health monitoring after nuclear accidents. IARC technical publication No.46. [internet, cited 2024 July 15] Available from: https://publications.iarc.fr/Book-And-Report-Series/Iarc-Technical-Publications/Thyroid-Health-Monitoring-After-Nuclear-Accidents-2018.
5. Miyauchi A, *et al.* Natural history of papillary thyroid microcarcinoma: kinetic analysis on tumor volume during active surveillance and before presentation. **Surgery** 165:25-30, 2019.
6. Hay ID, *et al.* Papillary thyroid carcinoma (PTC) in children and adults: Comparison of initial presentation and long-term postoperative outcome in 4432 patients consecutively treated at the Mayo Clinic during eight decades (1936–2015).

World J Surg 42:329–42, 2018.
7. Suzuki S. Management of thyroid cancer detected in heath checkup: Indication for operation. *Official Journal of the Japan Association of Endocrine Surgeons and the Japanese Society of Thyroid Surgery* 35:70-6, 2018 (in Japanese).
8. Shimura H. Evaluations and current issues for Thyroid Ultrasound Examination program in Fukushima Health Management Survey. *J Jpn Thyroid Assoc* 12:133-8, 2021 (in Japanese).
9. Suzuki S. Practice of surgical treatment for pediatric thyroid cancer in Fukushima Prefecture. *J Jpn Thyroid Assoc* 12:139-48, 2021 (in Japanese).
10. Science Council of Japan. Japan: Recommendations and reports (in Japanese). [internet, cited 2024 July 15] Available from: https://www.scj.go.jp/ja/info/kohyo/pdf/kohyo-23-h170901.pdf.
11. Takano T. Overdiagnosis of juvenile thyroid cancer. *Eur Thyroid J* 9:124-31, 2020.
12. Sakamoto A, *et al*. Cytological examination of the thyroid in children and adolescents after the Fukushima Nuclear Power Plant accident: the Fukushima Health Management Survey. *Endocr J* 67:1233-8, 2020.
13. Midorikawa S, Ohtsuru A. The impact of a misinterpretation of the term "overtreatment." *Endocr J* 67:1253-5, 2020.
14. Japan Thyroid Association. Thyroid cancer in children and adolescents found in the thyroid examination in the Fukushima Health Management Survey. In: Guidebook for Thyroid Specialists (2nd ed.). SHINDAN TO CHIRYO SYA Inc., pp.351-5, 2018 (in Japanese).
15. Rogers WA. Thyroid cancer overdiagnosis: the ethical issues. *J Jpn Thyroid Assoc* 12:16-21, 2021.
16. Takano T. Natural history of thyroid cancer : Self-limiting cancer as the cause of overdiagnosis. *J Jpn Thyroid Assoc* 12:22-7, 2021(in Japanese).
17. Ueno E. Impacts and adverse effects caused by the introduction of thyroid ultrasound -Pseudo endemic disease. *J Jpn Thyroid Assoc* 12:28-33, 2021(in Japanese).
18. Tsugane S. Radiation exposure and thyroid cancer after the Fukushima nuclear accident : The effect of overdiagnosis in causal relationship assessment. *J Jpn Thyroid Assoc* 12:45-51, 2021(in Japanese).
19. Ohtsuru A, Midorikawa S. Pros and cons of thyroid cancer screening after the nuclear accident : Focusing on recommendations from international agency and task force. *J Jpn Thyroid Assoc* 12:52-6, 2021(in Japanese).
20. Japan Thyroid Association. Japan: The opinion of the Japan Thyroid Association on

the special topic "Considering thyroid cancer overdiagnosis" published in Vol. 12, No. 1 of the Journal of the Japan Thyroid Association (in Japanese). [internet, cited 2024 July 15] Available from: https://www.japanthyroid.jp/public/img/news/20210609_1201_2_opinion.pdf.
21. Ohtsuru A. The occurrence and frequency of overdiagnosis/overtreatment cannot be evaluated by postoperative pathological findings or surgical procedures. *J Jpn Thyroid Assoc* 13:77, 2022 (in Japanese).
22. Ohtsuru A. Misleading overdiagnosis is a burden on residents and the affected society. *J Jpn Thyroid Assoc* 13:78, 2022 (in Japanese).
23. Suzuki S. Response to letters to the editor. *J Jpn Thyroid Assoc* 13:79-80, 2022 (in Japanese).
24. Shimura H. Response to letters to the editor. *J Jpn Thyroid Assoc* 13:81-2, 2022 (in Japanese).
25. Save Children from Overdiagnosis. Japan: Mamoru-chan digest in 5 minutes (in Japanese). [internet, cited 2024 July 15] Available from: https://www.youtube.com/watch?v=nY-AnZfT7b8.
26. Japan Consortium of Juvenile Thyroid Cancer. Japan: Thyroid Cancer Overdiagnosis 3-2: Use of social media. [internet, cited 2024 July 15] Available from: https://www.youtube.com/watch?v=F34i_O7G98k.
27. Save Children from Overdiagnosis. Japan: Save Children from Overdiagnosis on X (in Japanese). [internet, cited 2024 July 15] Available from: https://twitter.com/MKoujyo.
28. Japanese Association of Breast and Thyroid Sonology. Japan: Qualification certification for thyroid ultrasound-guided fine-needle aspiration cytology (in Japanese). [internet, cited 2024 July 15] Available from: https://jabts.jp/wp-content/uploads/2022/08/comittee12_2.pdf.
29. Japan Consortium of Juvenile Thyroid Cancer. Japan: About us. [internet, cited 2024 July 15] Available from: https://jcjtc.org/en/about-us/
30. Japan Consortium of Juvenile Thyroid Cancer. Japan: Thyroid Cancer Overdiagnosis: Voice from Fukushima 1. [internet, cited 2024 July 15] Available from: https://www.youtube.com/watch?v=-WxFCLqM1UQ.
31. Japan Consortium of Juvenile Thyroid Cancer. Japan: Thyroid Cancer Overdiagnosis: Voice from Fukushima 2. [internet, cited 2024 July 15] Available from: https://www.youtube.com/watch?v=NvAvvvbODW4.
32. Japan Consortium of Juvenile Thyroid Cancer. Japan: Thyroid Cancer Overdiagnosis: Round-table Discussion Part 1. [internet, cited 2024 March]

Available from: https://www.youtube.com/watch?v=9igUFg3k244.
33. Japan Consortium of Juvenile Thyroid Cancer. Japan: Thyroid Cancer Overdiagnosis: Round-table Discussion Part 2. [internet, cited 2024 July 15] Available from: https://www.youtube.com/watch?v=o1CK8n5_qr8.
34. Japan Consortium of Juvenile Thyroid Cancer. Japan: Thyroid Cancer Overdiagnosis 3-3: Opinion of an examinee. [internet, cited 2024 July 15] Available from: https://www.youtube.com/watch?v=7WsdED9LY0I.
35. Clero E, et al. Lessons learned from Chernobyl and Fukushima on thyroid cancer screening and recommendations in case of a future nuclear accident. *Environ Int* 146:106230, 2021.
36. Togawa K, et al. Long-term strategies for thyroid health monitoring after nuclear accidents: recommendations from an Expert Group convened by IARC. *Lancet Oncol* 19: 1280-3, 2018.
37. Liustko L, et al. The SHAMISEN recommendations on preparedness and health surveillance of populations affected by a radiation accident. *Environ Int* 146:106278, 2021.
38. UNSCEAR. Vienna, Austria: UNSCEAR 2020/2021 report volume II. [internet, cited 2024 July 15] Available from: https://www.unscear.org/unscear/publications/2020_2021_2.html.
39. Fukushima Medical University. Fukushima, Japan: 2021 Fukushima Medical University International Symposium on the Fukushima Health Management Survey. [internet, cited 2024 July 15] Available from: https://fhms.jp/symposium/uploads/symposium2021_02.pdf.
40. Fukushima Prefecture. Fukushima, Japan: The Prefectural Oversight Committee for the FHMS (in Japanese). [internet, cited 2024 July 15] Available from: https://www.pref.fukushima.lg.jp/site/portal/kenkocyosa-kentoiinkai.html.
41. Fukushima Prefecture. Fukushima, Japan: The Task Force for Thyroid Examination (in Japanese). [internet, cited 2024 July 15] Available from: https://www.pref.fukushima.lg.jp/sec/21045b/kenkocyosa-kentoiinkai-b.html.
42. Sakamoto A, et al. Overview of pathological diagnosis (cytology and histology) of the Fukushima Health Management Survey with a discussion of "overdiagnosis." *Official Journal of the Japan Association of Endocrine Surgeons and the Japanese Society of Thyroid Surgery* 39: 23-7, 2022 (in Japanese).

Chapter 6
Contributions of politicians, political activists, and the general public to the Fukushima overdiagnosis and overtreatment controversy

As a preamble to this chapter, the intention of this book is not to take sides in a political conflict but to educate readers. The authors believe that the thyroid examination in Fukushima needs major modifications if it is to continue. Participation must be completely voluntary, and survey participants must receive adequate information to improve health literacy, including a discussion of the survey's potential harms and benefits. The authors' goal is to help the children and young adults in Fukushima and the rest of Japan to lead healthy and happy lives. The objections to the thyroid ultrasound examination (TUE) expressed in this book have no basis in politics but in a sincere desire to prevent psychosocial and physical harm caused by cancer labeling, overdiagnosis and subsequent overtreatment.

Chapter 5 discusses the conflicts between physicians concerned about overdiagnosis and leadership members of the academic societies who support the thyroid examination in Fukushima. However, the controversy over the benefits and harms of the thyroid examination involves many different groups of people including not only physicians and radiation experts but also politicians, political activists, and Fukushima residents.

Many leadership members of the Fukushima Health Management Survey (FHMS) and some academic societies strongly support the continuation of the thyroid examination for reasons discussed previously. In addition, thyroid cancer diagnosis has been used as a powerful tool by anti-nuclear power activists to support their cause. Many individuals who lack expertise in medicine and thyroid neoplasia have become involved in the Fukushima TUE controversy, and their activities have had consequences. This chapter gives a detailed record of these individuals' activities and their consequences.

Section 1
Residents and citizen groups

Fukushima residents rarely mention concerns about the harm of overdiagnosis. The main reason is that they are not informed about the harmful effects of the thyroid examination.[1] The word "overdiagnosis" never appears in the bulletin distributed by Fukushima Prefecture explaining the ongoing thyroid examination (Table 4-3). A questionnaire survey of the residents showed that few know that a TUE can be harmful.[2, 3]

Most thyroid cancers diagnosed via ultrasound (US) screening are classical papillary thyroid carcinomas (PTC). Prior to the Fukushima thyroid examination, children, adolescents, and caregivers had not been given a detailed explanation of overdiagnosis, the self-limiting growth of most PTC, and the curability of nearly all PTC even if symptoms occur. Unfortunately, since a significant part of the thyroid examination is conducted under the guidance of schoolteachers, there is little chance for parents to ask questions. Thus, those diagnosed with thyroid cancer and their caregivers are likely to accept the statements by the Fukushima Prefecture that early diagnosis and surgical treatment will improve prognosis and quality of life (see Table 4-3).

The thyroid examination in Fukushima has become a tool for anti-nuclear energy groups. Its information is being actively disseminated by citizen groups campaigning against nuclear power. Their main claims are that the cases of thyroid cancer found in the FHMS were caused by radiation exposure, and the examination helps improve children's health and should be expanded. Reports of increasing cases of thyroid cancer and attribution of these cancers to radiation released during the nuclear power plant accident incite fear and further the argument for finding alternatives to nuclear energy. Opposition to the thyroid examination is being seen as an attempt to conceal the harms of the nuclear plant accident rather than an effort to allow children to live happy lives free of stress and stigma.

In addition to recommending against population screening, the International Agency for Cancer Research (IARC) stresses the need for voluntary participation and full informed consent when offering monitoring to high-risk groups.[4] Details of IARC recommendations and views of the leadership members of the FHMS are discussed in Chapters 4 and 5. *"Primum no nocere"* (first, do no harm) should be the motivation for opposition to mass thyroid US screening, not political views on nuclear energy.

As described in Chapter 4, some civic organizations voluntarily conduct thyroid US examinations for children and adolescents throughout Japan. Spokespeople for these organizations claim that they are testing outside Fukushima because not only Fukushima prefecture but all of Japan is polluted with radioactive substances. The examinations are justified by some thyroid specialists, including some chief members of thyroid-related academic societies, who state that there have been no overdiagnosed cases in Fukushima and that overdiagnosis will not occur as long as they strictly follow the Japanese guidelines.[5-7] Spokespersons also insist that the experts concerned about thyroid cancer overdiagnosis are involved in the interests of nuclear power plants.

In 2020, some thyroid specialists and Fukushima residents jointly established Preventing Overdiagnosis from Fukushima (POFF), a non-profit voluntary organization, to help people understand the thyroid examination correctly.[8] This organization publishes books, provides information through its homepage, holds study sessions through residents' representatives, and provides individual consultation and support by telephone or e-mail.[9]

In 2022, six patients diagnosed with thyroid cancer found in the FHMS sued the Tokyo Electric Power Company Holdings (TEPCO), which ran the Fukushima Daiichi nuclear power plant. The plaintiffs in this case are backed by lawyers who are deeply involved in the anti-nuclear movement. The plaintiffs claim they developed thyroid cancer because they were exposed to radiation from the nuclear plant accident. The lawyers in charge claim that some of these patients have metastases and recurrences, so there is no possibility of overdiagnosis. This claim is the same as that of the experts who favor continuing the examination. Their press conference was widely reported in newspapers and television throughout Japan. As a result, rumors have spread on social media and other media that children in Fukushima are more susceptible to thyroid cancer due to the damage caused by radiation exposure. Some even said that children in Fukushima are genetically polluted.

Such unfounded fears can be prevented from causing actual harm if the government and academic societies diligently publicize correct information, for example, the very low risk of radiation-induced thyroid carcinomas and the increasing risk of overdiagnosis and overtreatment in Fukushima. However, their response was slow and limited. They might fear that emphasizing such information might trigger criticism of the FHMS.

Reports linking the nuclear plant accident to the occurrence of thyroid cancer in Fukushima were seen not only in Japan but also in overseas media, such as the British Broadcasting Corporation (BBC).

Section 2
The politicians weigh in

In 2016, the Fukushima Pediatric Association submitted a request for a reduction of the thyroid examination to Fukushima Prefecture. The request pointed out that the large number of thyroid cancers found in the examination so far had caused health concerns for Fukushima's children, parents, and citizens. The submitted document requested reconsideration of the examination, including a review of the methods of diagnosis and subsequent surgery. However, this request received fierce protests from some citizen groups who claimed that a reduction in the scale of the thyroid examination goes against the medical principle of "early detection and early treatment." As a result, no subsequent requests have been made by the association. On the other hand, a petition was submitted to the Fukushima Prefectural Assembly by a citizen group to maintain the scale of- and easy access to the thyroid examination and to disseminate correct information. This petition was unanimously adopted.

It is only recently that the harmful effects of overdiagnosis associated with the thyroid examination in Fukushima have been regarded as a social problem by national and prefectural parliaments. In 2020, Shun Otokita, a member of the House of Councilors, first took up this issue in the Diet, followed by Kohei Watanabe, who first took it up in the Fukushima Prefectural Assembly. After that, Goshi Hosono, the Minister of the Environment at the time of the Great East Japan Earthquake and one of the people in charge of starting the thyroid examination in Fukushima, pointed out the problem of overdiagnosis to the Diet members. However, the opinions of these individuals did not bring about change to the FHMS because the concerns about overdiagnosis were voiced by a minority of assembly members. Fukushima Prefecture and the Ministry of the Environment did not officially admit the existence of harm from overdiagnosis. On the contrary, some politicians repeatedly accused the government of not admitting that radiation is causing thyroid cancer in Fukushima. They called for further expansion of the thyroid examination.

One of the reasons why politicians who point out the problem of the thyroid examination in Fukushima remain in the minority is that the general public finds it difficult to accept the claim that overdiagnosis is a problem. Rather than calling out the risk of overdiagnosis, the claim that the thyroid examination should be continued and expanded to protect children's health seems more common sense. Moreover, in Japan, not a few experts, mainly senior academics, still deny the harm of overdiagnosis related to the thyroid examination. Thus, it is considered that opinions are still divided among experts. From these, it is likely that they do not want to take the risk of pointing out the problem of overdiagnosis and incurring the backlash of their supporters.

In January 2022, five former Japanese Prime Ministers sent a letter to the European Union (EU) Secretariat against the EU's decision to make nuclear power an environmentally friendly method of power generation.[10] Many people have questioned the statement in their letter that stated, "Children in Fukushima are suffering from thyroid cancer due to the nuclear accident." There was fierce criticism of the former ministers' letter by those who doubted the relationship between Fukushima's cases of thyroid cancer and radiation. This criticism was reported by mass media and attracted the attention of the general public.

The Fukushima Prefecture and the Ministry of the Environment of Japan immediately expressed opposition to this letter. The content of the 2020 United Nations Scientific Committee on the Effects of Atomic Radiation (UNSCEAR) report was the basis for their opposition.[11] The UNSCEAR report arrives at two conclusions. One is that the thyroid cancer found in Fukushima is not being caused by radiation exposure, and the other is that overdiagnosis may be occurring. The Fukushima Prefecture emphasized the conclusion that radiation is not the cause of Fukushima thyroid carcinoma. However, although overdiagnosis would explain why so many Fukushima children are being diagnosed with thyroid cancer, they do not mention the possible overdiagnosis part. The Minister of the Environment was asked by a newspaper reporter how to tackle the problem of overdiagnosis. He refused to answer, saying, "It is none of my business."

As can be seen from the above paragraphs, the use of the TUE findings in the FHMS and avoidance of discussion of overdiagnosis have become political issues rather than solely medical concerns.

Section 3 Media and publishers

There is a big difference in media coverage between the central national and Fukushima local news media. Neither, however, are very keen on reporting about thyroid cancer overdiagnosis. The main concern of central media coverage is the number of patients with thyroid cancer found in the FHMS. Several press releases reported the results of the FHMS in a manner to suggest that radiation exposure was causing the increased numbers of patients with thyroid cancer and that early diagnosis and treatment in Fukushima help protect children's health. Again, there were reports that experts were using concern for overdiagnosis to conceal health damage caused by the nuclear power plant accident.

A typical example is a 2022 news program broadcasted on Tokyo Broadcasting System Television (TBS), one of the central Japanese television stations. The show included a detailed report about the Fukushima thyroid cancer patients who sued TEPCO. During this program, the following was conveyed: First, thyroid cancer in Fukushima is likely to be caused by radiation from the nuclear plant accident, and second, Fukushima Prefecture claims that the cause of thyroid cancer is overdiagnosis. Neither of these messages is accurate. The intention of TBS was likely to convince viewers that the nuclear accident is causing health hazards that are being concealed by the Fukushima Prefecture via the promotion of overdiagnosis as the cause of cancer diagnoses. A Japanese epidemiologist, who claims that thyroid cancer in Fukushima is being caused by radiation exposure, was the only expert to appear on the program.[12]

The Fukushima local media was relatively balanced its reporting. While the health effects of radiation were not over-reported, there were few in-depth discussions of the health hazards caused by the thyroid examination. No report has criticized Fukushima Prefecture or the Japanese government for ignoring the harm of overdiagnosis. This absence of criticism may reflect the trust and regard that Fukushima residents have for the Fukushima experts, especially those at Fukushima Medical University (FMU). Residents and local media respect the FMU experts, who are different from those promoting the TUE, but when the FMU is promoting the thyroid examination, residents won't know the difference. Expert opinions for and against the TUE are thrown at readers without any in-depth discussion of the meaning and causes of overdiagnosis and its harms.

A dedicated effort is now being made to educate both the Japanese and overseas public by using the Internet to disseminate information in both Japanese and English. This effort is intended to help both the residents of Fukushima and others to understand the reasons that some experts see the thyroid examination as harmful. Misaki Hattori, editor-in-chief of the Fukushima Report, was helping with this educational program. Hattori had collaborated with several experts from Japan and around the world to inform the public about the thyroid examination in Fukushima. Those interviewed by Hattori include world-renowned experts such as Hyeong Sik Ahn (Korea University, South Korea) and Louise Davies (Geisel School of Medicine at Dartmouth, U.S.A.).[13, 14]

The editors-in-chief of Japanese academic journals usually have leadership roles in associated academic societies. These societies have shown little interest in addressing thyroid cancer overdiagnosis in Fukushima. Thus, there have been few publications dealing with thyroid cancer overdiagnosis in Japanese academic journals. However, there are now signs of change. In 2021, an academic publisher, Igaku-shoin (Tokyo, Japan), addressed the issue of thyroid cancer overdiagnosis in its weekly newspaper. This publication became one of the most visited articles in 2021.[15] Shinichi Okabayashi, the president of a new publishing company, Akebishobo (Tokyo), regards thyroid cancer overdiagnosis in Fukushima as a severe social problem and decided to publish a book on this problem. The first book on thyroid cancer in Fukushima, co-authored by five experts, was published in 2021.[16]

In 2023, manga artist Yoko Hano began serializing a manga called "It's painful when my first love keeps flagging with my brother." Some episodes depict a harsh criticism of the FHMS.[17] The heroine was diagnosed with thyroid cancer in the thyroid examination, and she is now followed up without surgery. In other words, she is an overdiagnosed case. The description of her health condition in this manga uses the term "overdiagnosis," and it explains that "Early detection of thyroid cancer through screening is not internationally recommended." Both of these are that Fukushima Prefecture and FMU have avoided explaining to the residents of Fukushima. It also provides harsh criticism, saying, "There is no way that the doctors who launched the thyroid examination would admit that the examination is harmful." and "She is a victim of an unnecessary examination." The author is a resident of Fukushima Prefecture, and the story conveys the anger of the people of Fukushima towards the prefecture and FMU conducting the thyroid examination without honestly telling the people about the reality of the examination. A spinoff of this manga, "A Scary Story from an Endocrinologist," was posted on X in June 2024 and received two million views in one day.[18]

References

1. Japan Consortium of Juvenile Thyroid Cancer. Japan: Thyroid Cancer Overdiagnosis: Voice from Fukushima 1. [internet, cited 2024 July 15] Available from: https://www.youtube.com/watch?v=-WxFCLqM1UQ.
2. Fukushima Prefecture. Fukushima, Japan: Results of interviews with subjects undergoing thyroid examination (in Japanese). [internet, cited 2024 July 15] Available from: https://www.pref.fukushima.lg.jp/uploaded/attachment/446631.pdf.
3. Fukushima Report. Japan: What are the risks and benefits of Fukushima's thyroid examination? (in Japanese) [internet, cited 2024 July 15] Available from:

https://synodos.jp/fukushima-report/22520/
4. International Agency for Research on Cancer. Lyon, France: Thyroid health monitoring after nuclear accidents. IARC technical publication No.46. [internet, cited 2024 July 15] Available from: https://publications.iarc.fr/Book-And-Report-Series/Iarc-Technical-Publications/Thyroid-Health-Monitoring-After-Nuclear-Accidents-2018.
5. Suzuki S. Management of thyroid cancer detected in heath checkup: Indication for operation. *Official Journal of the Japan Association of Endocrine Surgeons and the Japanese Society of Thyroid Surgery* 35:70-6, 2018 (in Japanese).
6. Shimura H. Evaluations and current issues for Thyroid Ultrasound Examination program in Fukushima Health Management Survey. *J Jpn Thyroid Assoc* 12:133-8, 2021 (in Japanese).
7. Suzuki S. Practice of surgical treatment for pediatric thyroid cancer in Fukushima Prefecture. *J Jpn Thyroid Assoc* 12:139-48, 2021 (in Japanese).
8. Preventing Overdiagnosis from Fukushima. Japan: POFF (in Japanese). [internet, cited 2024 July 15] Available from: https://www.poff-jp.com.
9. Ohtsuru A, Midorikawa S. Michishirube. POFF, 2020 (in Japanese).
10. Japan Times. Tokyo, Japan: Ex-prime ministers Koizumi and Kan demand EU choose zero nuclear power path. [internet, cited 2024 July 15] Available from: https://www.japantimes.co.jp/news/2022/01/27/national/koizumi-kan-nuclear/.
11. UNSCEAR. Vienna, Austria: UNSCEAR 2020/2021 report volume II. [internet, cited 2024 July 15] Available from: https://www.unscear.org/unscear/publications/2020_2021_2.html.
12. Tsuda T, et al. Thyroid cancer detection by ultrasound among residents ages 18 years and younger in Fukushima, Japan: 2011 to 2014. *Epidemiology* 27:316-22, 2016.
13. Fukushima Report. Japan: Conveying Korean's lessons to Fukushima: Overdiagnosis of thyroid cancer in Korea and the thyroid examination in Fukushima (in Japanese). [internet, cited 2024 July 15] Available from: https://synodos.jp/fukushima-report/21930/.
14. Fukushima Report. Japan: How to make use of IARC recommendation for Fukushima. [internet, cited 2024 July 15] Available from: https://synodos.jp/fukushima-report/23001/.
15. Igaku-shoin. Japan: Takano T, *et a l*. Eliminate the number of people who become unhappy due to overdiagnosis: From the lessons of the Fukushima nuclear accident (in Japanese). [internet, cited 2024 July 15] Available from:

https://www.igaku-shoin.co.jp/paper/archive/y2021/3408_01.
16. Takano T, et al. Thyroid examination and overdiagnosis in Fukushima: What can we do for the children? Akebishobo, 2021 (in Japanese).
17. Hano Y. It's painful when my first love keeps flagging with my brother. Volumes 1-3. Koudansha, 2024 (in Japanese).
18. Hano Y. A Scary Story from an Endocrinologist (in Japanese). [internet, cited 2024 July 15] Available from: https://note.com/hnyk0720/n/n233df8f5a1f1.

Chapter 7
Personal perspectives of physicians directly involved in the Fukushima thyroid ultrasound examination

Chapters 5 and 6 discussed the views and activities of academics and their respective societies, politicians, political activists, and journalism. Chapter 7 provides a detailed, chronological account of the personal experiences of two physicians directly involved in the thyroid examination in Fukushima and the thoughts of two others affected by the program. Some of the material has been previously discussed; however, in this chapter, readers will be given insight into the Fukushima thyroid examination controversy from the personal perspectives of those directly involved in the program.

The thyroid examination, including a thyroid ultrasound examination (TUE) for the Fukushima Health Management Survey (FHMS), began as a large-scale screening project for thyroid cancer involving approximately 380,000 young people. It was initiated in October 2011, just six months after the nuclear accident, and the thyroid examination has been ongoing for more than thirteen years. During the early stages of the thyroid examination, Drs. Sanae Midorikawa and Akira Ohtsuru had been responsible members of the staff at Fukushima Medical University (FMU) and were involved in the day-to-day operations of the program. In this chapter, Drs. Midorikawa and Ohtsuru describe the events that occurred and their thoughts during this period.

They explain why the thyroid examination was initiated and how concerns for overdiagnosis and patient harm arose. These concerns led to conflicts, some of which have been described in previous chapters. The personal stories of the physicians who participated actively in the thyroid examination are told in this chapter, allowing readers to compare the views of those working directly with children in the thyroid examination with those from outside.

Section 1
Start-up of the thyroid examination from the perspective of a medical doctor in Fukushima

1. **Situation before the thyroid examination and implementation of a new screening program (2011)**

   Dr. Sanae Midorikawa, one of the authors, is a medical doctor and endocrinologist who was a member of the FMU faculty at the time of the Great East Japan earthquake and the nuclear plant accident. In June 2011, she heard the news that a thyroid examination was about to begin. Since thyroid disease is part of her specialty in endocrine disorders, she wanted to contribute to the thyroid examination and help alleviate the anxiety of children and caregivers in Fukushima. The residents, particularly mothers, were concerned about thyroid disease due to radiation exposure. Her colleagues, acquaintances, and friends with children often asked her, "Are the children's thyroid glands in Fukushima safe? Will it be like Chornobyl?" As a doctor specializing in endocrine disorders in Fukushima, she felt compelled to contribute to the thyroid examination. No one could accurately predict the outcome of this examination, and few expressed concerns about initiating a screening program without prior evidence regarding benefits and harms. She and other doctors in Fukushima believed that the thyroid examination would provide reassurance and confidence, especially to many mothers.

   In September 2011, during a television interview after an international conference following the Fukushima nuclear power plant accident, the newly appointed director of the Radiation Medical Science Center at FMU announced, "Decision has been made to conduct a thyroid examination. This will be the first large-scale survey in the world." At this point, the details of the thyroid examination had not yet been decided, and even Midorikawa, who would be on the front lines of the examination, had no information about what would happen next. A commission of FHMS experts started discussing how to conduct the thyroid examination.

   Initially, Midorikawa was not a member of this committee but joined after the examination started. Her supervisor at that time, a professor in the Department of Diabetes, Endocrinology, and Metabolism, was one of the original members of the committee. He occasionally consulted Midorikawa about the planning of the TUE, asking questions such as, "Can you examine babies?" "How many children can you examine per day?" He was skeptical about thyroid cancer screening in children due to a lack of clear evidence of benefits and was not eager to support it. As a result, he decided not to provide staff from his department for the TUE actively. Therefore, Midorikawa and another endocrinologist volunteered to participate in the TUE using time outside of their regular clinical practices and teaching duties.

In October 2011, Dr. Akira Ohtsuru, a physician with expertise in the care of atomic bomb survivors and radiation health risk sciences, was invited to FMU as a professor in the Department of Radiation Health Management from Nagasaki University and joined the commission of experts. At that time, the principal policy for the thyroid examination had already been decided, but the details were unclear, and no one was sure which survey method would be the best.

Ohtsuru provided health consultations to over 1,000 people in six months following the nuclear plant accident. He felt that the residents' concerns about thyroid cancer were strong, and addressing these concerns was necessary. Many people requested a whole-body counter (WBC) examination to evaluate their internal radiation exposure. As a result of this examination, it became evident that the internal exposure doses were so low that they would not be expected to affect the thyroid or health in general. Of note, while the people who came for consultation had vague concerns, they did not specifically express a desire for an ultrasound (US) examination.

2. How the thyroid US examination was initiated (2011-2013)

As discussed in Chapter 2, the examination consists of two parts: the primary TUE and the confirmatory examination, as defined by the protocol.[1] If primary US shows no cysts or nodules, cysts ≤ 20mm, or nodules ≤ 5mm, subjects are scheduled for follow-up US in 2 years. If larger cysts or nodules are found, the examinee is referred for a more detailed confirmatory examination with a recommendation for fine-needle aspiration cytology (FNAC) if confirmatory examination findings deem cytological evaluation necessary. The thyroid examination was started in October 2011. During the first month, it was conducted at FMU partly as a test run. The first group of subjects was examined at FMU. During the next month, a team consisting of doctors, medical technologists, nurses, and FMU office workers visited communities to conduct the examination. A meeting for the evaluation of the US images was set up at FMU, and the results of the primary examination were returned to the examinees. After the evaluation of the primary examination results, the confirmatory examination, called the secondary examination, was begun. Many people were concerned about the results. Later, cases of thyroid carcinoma or suspicious for thyroid carcinoma were found via the confirmatory examination.

According to the original FHMS plan, the first round of the thyroid examination was to be conducted for two and a half years, from October 2011 to March 2014.[2] The target population consisted of approximately 360,000 individuals, so the plan for the TUE was based on the estimate that about 750 children would be examined per day in order to complete the first-round examination within the allotted time frame. In order to handle such a large number of examinations, examinations during school classes started in November 2011. The FMU staff, including Midorikawa and Ohtsuru, admit that school examinations were initiated partly for the convenience of the organizers of the TUE, as it allowed for more efficient planning. Especially in the early years, there was a shortage of medical staff to conduct US examinations. Even with the cooperation of doctors, clinical technologists, and radiologists from all over Japan who were familiar with thyroid US, FMU struggled to secure enough personnel to conduct US examinations on any given day.

In January 2012, Midorikawa moved within the university to the Department of Radiation Health Management and started to work with Ohtsuru and other staff members in the Department. Midorikawa began to spend 3-4 days a week going out for US examinations. The US examiners were required to work efficiently in order to complete all the scheduled examinations for the day. Children and caregivers who came for the TUE appeared to be very anxious. For many people, this was their first time experiencing a thyroid US examination. They were anxious about the examination itself. Would it be painful? Mothers with small children were also concerned about whether their children could take the examination. They did not understand the purpose of the TUE nor that the first round (baseline survey) was being performed earlier than the expected onset of detectable radiation-induced thyroid cancers (4-5 years post-exposure).

Mothers worried that radiation-induced cancer might already be present in their children's thyroid glands and incorrectly believed that a TUE could determine radiation exposure levels. During the first round of the thyroid examination, examiners were often asked by examinees or their caretakers about the "radiation dose." They did not understand that a TUE could not predict the level of radiation exposure or dose absorbed. At first, the examiners were not allowed to explain the results to the examinees immediately after the US study. Some doctors would explain, if asked; however, discussing results with examinees required extra time and had the potential to prevent completion of all the day's scheduled examinations.

A cancer diagnosis is made at the confirmatory examination step. During 2012 and 2013, the number of cancer diagnoses was small because the confirmatory examination was not yet advanced. No one knew the number that would be eventually diagnosed.

Therefore, the issue of overdiagnosis and the related psychosocial problems had not yet arisen at that time. The most pressing concern was how to provide timely and better explanations to the examinees. The confusion and anxiety caused by the TUE classifications, including the "A2 problem," is discussed in Chapter 3. The TUE project team's policy at that time prioritized a smooth and efficient examination process over addressing the concerns of the examinees. As a result, it was not possible to immediately implement a system that provided thorough explanations, even at public facilities where both examinees and their caregivers were present.

During this period, risk communication following the nuclear accident was not effective. The public did not trust the government's announcements, opinions on radiation exposure, or the thyroid examination being conducted by the FHMS. Some examinees complained that they were suffering from the effects of radiation exposure, and some parents blamed the person in charge of the examination site for flaws in the examination system. It was inevitable that some staff members would want to escape from these unpleasant situations. It was difficult for the staff to respond to the residents' concerns or reassure them there was nothing to worry about. The inability to explain the results was stressful for the staff. Thus, the examination venue did not allow for individual questions to be addressed during the TUE.

This raises questions about the ethicality of the screening program in which participants' and caregivers' questions or concerns cannot be addressed prior to participation. FMU, the Fukushima Prefecture, or the Prefectural Oversight Committee for the FHMS (POCF) focused on the efficiency and participation rate of the screening rather than these ethical issues in the initial phase. This seems to be one of the reasons why no one had any doubts about thyroid examinations being carried out as part of school examinations.

The examiners routinely take several US images per person at the examination site as a record. If a nodule of any size is found, the examiner makes video images for the record so that the expert panel can later distinguish between nodules with benign features (categories A1, A2) and those requiring further work-up and FNAC (category B). Therefore, a large number of images are accumulated daily. The officers and medical staff of the Radiation Medical Science Center organized the examination report forms with images and findings, and a meeting with several experts is held weekly to check and classify the images into categories of A1, A2, and B. [1]

After US interpretive decisions are made, results are mailed to each examinee, along with a brief explanation of the meaning of the result. However, as explained in Chapter 3, people who received an A2 or B result became very anxious, and the call center of the Radiation Medical Science Center at FMU received numerous phone inquiries about A2 and sometimes B results. There were many questions that physicians should have answered directly, but they were unable to respond adequately immediately after the examination. As discussed in Chapter 3, even cysts and nodules of no medical significance caused great concern among examinees and their parents. Some thyroid specialists argued that a standardized system based on clinical guidelines could prevent confusion. However, Midorikawa and Ohtsuru believe that inadequate explanations led to residents' concerns about the examination results and caused anxiety and distrust of FMU and the Fukushima Prefecture.[3,4]

3. Thyroid cancers were found in the confirmatory examination (2012-2014)

As the TUE progressed, the number of examinees receiving a result of category B increased gradually. The study protocol required that Category B, defined as nodule > 5 mm or cyst > 20 mm, must have additional US study to determine the need for FNAC. Thus, the confirmatory examination is performed on examinees with Category B nodules or cysts. The confirmatory examination began long after the screening examination. Initially, only one doctor was involved, so it took more than six months for subjects to receive detailed examination reports. The director of the department of TUE at that time explained that there was no need to rush because thyroid nodules progress slowly, even if they are cancerous. However, although thyroid specialists are aware of the benign or indolent nature of most thyroid nodules, the concept of indolent cancer is not broadly appreciated by the general public. Those who received a Category B result experienced long-term anxiety. Recognizing this situation, Midorikawa sometimes visited the confirmatory examination venue and spoke with examinees and their caregivers immediately after their examinations. She realized that the thyroid examination system, including the confirmatory examination, did not always provide peace of mind.

The confirmatory examination confirmed thyroid cancer in some young people, and the number of FNAC-detected thyroid cancers increased as the examination progressed. The results of the primary and confirmatory examinations were reported at a weekly commission meeting at the FMU. Experts attending the meeting recognized that thyroid cancer cases were being found one after another. They had anticipated that US screening of children and young adults, which had not been previously performed, could increase the detection rate of thyroid cancer to some extent. However, none of the experts involved in the thyroid screening in Fukushima predicted that more than 100 thyroid cancers would be detected by FNAC following the first round of screening. The thyroid specialists who were not involved in the TUE were also surprised by the number of cancers found, dozens of times higher than expected.

This surprise increased when the second round of screening also found thyroid cancer in people who had no abnormal findings in the first round examination performed two years earlier. At FMU meetings, some asked for the reason for these new cases, but no one could give a clear explanation. Midorikawa and Ohtsuru thought that overdiagnosis was a possibility, even in children and young adults. However, this idea was dismissed by the head of the TUE and some thyroid specialists who thought that overdiagnosis in children was impossible, even with US screening. The concept that self-limiting, harmless "cancers" develop in children could not be accepted by the TUE leadership (see Chapters 1 and 4).

Announcements to the residents about the results of the thyroid examination including the number of thyroid cancers, were given at the POCF meetings held approximately every three months, and the media reported on them. The number of thyroid cancer cases was regularly reported in the media, and the residents began to wonder if the increasing number of thyroid cancers was due to radiation exposure. At the TUE explanatory meetings given to the residents, more and more questions and concerns about thyroid cancer were raised. Those concerned about the health effects of radiation exposure said that the situation in Fukushima is the same as had occurred in Chornobyl. Those who were initially convinced that radiation exposure was low changed their minds and said that the reassurance that there was nothing to worry about was a lie. Some of them developed new fears that they or their families might develop thyroid cancer.[5]

It is impossible to determine the causal relationship between thyroid cancer and radiation dose in individual cases, and information released to the public is based on epidemiological analysis.[6] However, it was difficult for many residents to understand this. When radiation epidemiological results were explained, some claimed that the results of the thyroid examination were unreliable and even said that they were being treated like experimental guinea pigs. This confusion increased their risk perception of thyroid cancer. People often asked Midorikawa and Ohtsuru why the same examination was not being conducted outside of Fukushima Prefecture in order to see how Fukushima US findings compare to other prefectures. The reason why a large-scale thyroid examination has not been conducted outside of Fukushima as a control is that such a study has a risk of harm but no health benefits to subjects. However, the general public is not familiar with the concept of overdiagnosis, and it is difficult for people to understand why screening asymptomatic children with no risk factors can cause harm and could be considered unethical.

4. Efforts to lessen thyroid examination-related anxiety (2015)

Many doctors in Fukushima participated in the project because they believed the thyroid examination would address residents' concerns about children's health and relieve anxiety. Ironically, as discussed previously, this population-based survey led to increased anxiety. Even benign results, such as small cysts or A2 nodules, caused caregiver guilt and self-condemnation. Of course, detection of thyroid cancers reinforced anxiety about radiation exposure and the perceived increased risk of radiation-induced cancer.

In April 2015, when Midorikawa and Ohtsuru became involved in the operation of the thyroid examination, they implemented activities designed to explain the examination and prevent or at least lessen the program-related anxiety. They held explanatory meetings for the residents, on-site classes for children who were subjects of the thyroid examination, set up face-to-face counseling to explain the result immediately after the examination, and established a support system for the examinees and caretakers during the prolonged survey period. [3, 4]

Outsiders need to recognize that the Great East Japan earthquake and subsequent tsunami themselves caused an enormous amount of trauma and stress for Fukushima residents. Evacuations alone traumatized the residents, and the disruption of healthcare systems had an adverse effect on the elderly.[7] The thyroid examination placed additional stress on the examinees and their families. Some of these already traumatized residents said hurtful things to the staff who were trying to reduce anxiety via scientific explanations. Thus, some staff members became discouraged that their efforts did not seem to reduce anxiety, and the work was mentally draining. Midorikawa encouraged her colleagues to try to understand the residents' anxiety, even when vague, and attempt to address it. Some of the staff members were also earthquake victims, yet they did their best to help and support Fukushima residents.

5. Thoughts of an expert who led the thyroid examination: Dr. Shigenobu Nagataki

Anyone who has learned enough about the effects of radiation after the Chornobyl nuclear plant accident and dropping of the atomic bombs can understand that the high incidence of thyroid cancer in Fukushima was not caused by radiation. The exposure doses in Fukushima were far lower than those following the Chornobyl accident and the atomic bombings in Hiroshima and Nagasaki and are considered to be too low to present risk of thyroid cancer. However, it is important for the experts in charge to understand that demonstrating the scientific rationale for this fact is not enough to ease the residents' concerns.

The late Dr. Shigenobu Nagataki was Japan's leading expert on thyroid research and radiation effects, and he was deeply moved by the suffering of Fukushima residents. Midorikawa introduced Dr. Nagataki in an essay published on the website of the Japan Consortium of Juvenile Thyroid Cancer (JCJTC).[8]

Will of Dr. Nagataki
Sanae Midorikawa
Professor, Miyagi Gakuin Women's University

I first met the late Dr. Shigenobu Nagataki, a well-known expert in thyroidology and the health effects of radiation, at an international conference three years after the Fukushima nuclear accident. Dr. Akira Ohtsuru, who was once a graduate student and on the medical staff of Dr. Nagataki, introduced me as a chief doctor on the thyroid examination scene. At that time, the first round of thyroid examination had been completed, and the second round was ongoing. The number of thyroid cancers in children was increasing rapidly. This renewed the anxiety of many Fukushima residents who believed that they were experiencing the health effects of radiation.

Dr. Nagataki, an expert on both radiation and the thyroid, assured me that it was unlikely to be the effect of radiation. Thus, I could explain this to the residents with confidence. After that, I had few opportunities to talk directly with him. However, from time to time, he emailed Dr. Ohtsuru. He let us know about some critical academic papers and his interpretation of the data. Furthermore, he sent us and let us read his book, "Health Effects of Radiation Learned from Nuclear Disasters and Countermeasures," which was published very early after the nuclear accident (January 2012).

I would like to introduce some comments from Chapter 8 in this book, 'The protection, relief and assistance of the exposed people' as below. "Unregulated health examinations only increase the psychological distress of the survivors. Even when the survivors are free to take general medical check-ups, they are still worried because every time they find an abnormality, they regard it as the consequence of radiation exposure. Before starting a health survey, we should examine past disaster cases (including not only nuclear disasters but also other natural disasters). We should plan carefully so that we can clarify the purpose of the survey and the survey contributes to the true welfare of the people." He wrote about the health survey on the Fukushima nuclear accident as follows. *"It might be recommended to carry out a health examination in consideration of psychological aspects. However, based on the experience of disaster cases so far, the survey should be carefully planned so as not to promote further anxiety."* I read it again and was impressed by the fact that Dr. Nagataki foresaw the survey's negative effect, even before the thyroid examination was started.

In September 2016, two months before Dr. Nagataki died, the 5th Fukushima International Expert Meeting on Thyroid Cancer after the Nuclear Accident was held in Fukushima. Dr. Nagataki gave a keynote speech entitled *"Nagasaki University: 30 Years after the Chornobyl Accident: Contribution from Japan."* He talked about his involvement as a thyroid expert after the Chornobyl accident and cooperation with international organizations such as the IAEA and WHO.

In this meeting, Dr. Ohtsuru gave an overview of the results of the thyroid examination, and as a member of Fukushima Medical University, reported that overdiagnosis had occurred, for the first time at an international conference. Also, I presented some problems in the thyroid examination: 1) The results of the examination was causing new anxiety, 2) false-positive results and overdiagnosis were occurring as disadvantages of the thyroid cancer screening, leading to psycho-social problems, and 3) the survey was carried out in a semi-enforced manner.

At that time, Dr. Nagataki had health issues making it difficult to walk. When my presentation was over, and I got off the podium, he, who was sitting in the front row, bothered to stand up with the support of his wife and spoke to me. He praised me and said that he was much impressed by my presentation. Furthermore, in the general discussion the next day, he made a statement that the thyroid examination should not be continued in its current manner if it had been started only to deal with anxiety. When I met him again at the meeting of Japan Thyroid Association a few days before he died, I had some time to talk with him. He said that after listening to my presentation, he realized that the scientific facts do not directly lead to the peace of mind of the residents, and he hoped he would make an effort to modify the survey so that it would genuinely benefit Fukushima residents and give them confidence.

I have always cherished these words and take them as the will of Prof Nagataki. Dr. Nagataki was the leading expert in the contribution at Chornobyl and might have been one of the heroes in Chornobyl in a sense. However, he understood the truth about Chornobyl and the pain of the residents. He did not become a hero in Fukushima. I believe he was always thinking about what was necessary for

Fukushima residents.

Since he had a strong influence on the government, I think that if Dr. Nagataki were still alive, the thyroid examination would not be as it is now. I would like to consider again what we should do to meet the expectations of Dr. Nagataki.

Section 2
Confronting the problem of overdiagnosis and subsequent efforts to resolve it

1. Overdiagnosis was first pointed out in Fukushima (2014)

As described in Chapter 4, overdiagnosis regarding the thyroid examination in Fukushima was first pointed out publicly in March 2014 at a meeting of the Task Force for Thyroid Examination (TFTE) by Kenji Shibuya (University of Tokyo).[9] In May 2014, Shibuya et al. published a letter article in the Lancet in which the authors pointed out that both overdiagnosis and overtreatment were possible.[10] The authors stated that reconsideration of the Fukushima thyroid screening program is needed in order to reduce residents' fear and anxiety and the current program is unsuitable to evaluate for the effects of radiation or to ameliorate anxiety.

At the meeting, Yoshikazu Nishi (Hiroshima Red Cross Hospital), a pediatrician, introduced the fact that in some previous studies, many asymptomatic thyroid cancers were detected during thyroid gland palpation among university students and pointed out the possibility that high-precision US screening could result in the diagnosis of a large number of thyroid cancers.[11] Shoichiro Tsugane (National Cancer Center) presented documents on epidemiological findings regarding thyroid cancer screening and explained overdiagnosis.[12] He also explained the history of overdiagnosis of neuroblastoma, mass screening for children conducted in Japan, and its discontinuation due to overdiagnosis, as well as the problem of thyroid cancer screening in South Korea. In November 2014, a well-known article about the massive overdiagnosis occurring in South Korea due to thyroid cancer screening by Ahn et al. was published in the New England Journal of Medicine.[13]

The TFTE discussed this issue several times. At that time, Midorikawa and Ohtsuru were not responsible for TUE and did not participate in this committee. Members who participated on behalf of FMU responded to this concern by saying that they had already anticipated the possibility of overdiagnosis and had considered diagnostic criteria to prevent it as much as possible. In hindsight, this was not a valid answer to the problem of overdiagnosis, but profound study and productive discussion of the problem have not occurred. Instead, discussions have focused on how to explore the health effects of radiation exposure and how to offer the examination to the concerned residents.

Although there was a vague concern that the examination might be causing something terrible, this concern did not lead to a discussion about modifying the survey methods. There was insufficient discussion about whether overdiagnosis was occurring and to what extent. Overdiagnosis concerns were treated as irreconcilable with the need to continue the survey, which examines radiation effects. The opinions of TFTE members concerned about overdiagnosis are supported by previously cited scientific reports and outside experts' opinions; however, FMU and the Fukushima Prefecture interpreted overdiagnosis concerns as criticism of the university and prefecture officials rather than an effort to minimize harm.

Midorikawa and Ohtsuru had expected that a scientific analysis of the first round of the examination would indicate the possibility of overdiagnosis in the thyroid examination and motivate FHMS officials to take action against it. However, no such action was taken. Results of the first-round (baseline) examination were published in 2016.[1] The scientific benefits of acquiring data on the prevalence of colloid cysts and the baseline prevalence of small thyroid cancers were discussed in this paper; however, due to disagreement between the authors concerning the discussion of overdiagnosis, neither the possibility of overdiagnosis nor the potential negative psychologic effects of detecting harmless colloid cysts were addressed.

In 2014, the TFTE evaluated the results of the first-round examination. During this process, the results of the second-round examination were beginning to become public. The second round began to discover several thyroid cancers in people with no significant findings in the first round. By giving the impression that cancer is growing rapidly, not very slowly, these second-round findings have been used to support the cause of social activist groups against the use of nuclear energy. As discussed in Chapter 6, these groups have fiercely criticized experts' views that the thyroid examination survey is leading to the harm of overdiagnosis. These experts have been accused of concealing the harmful effects of radiation in Fukushima. This criticism may have significantly influenced the positions of Fukushima Prefecture, the Ministry of the Environment, and FMU.

The minutes of the expert meetings in Fukushima, such as those of the TFTE, clearly show that there is widespread misunderstanding of the definition of the term "overdiagnosis". As discussed in Chapter 1, the definition of overdiagnosis has recently been fixed. Cancer overdiagnosis is now used for patients who receive a correct pathologic diagnosis based on morphologic criteria; however, this "cancer," if never diagnosed, would not cause morbidity or mortality during the patient's lifetime. Admittedly, the concept of overdiagnosis is complex. Many people, both health professionals and the general public, do not understand the current usage. In fact, experts are still struggling to clarify its definition.[14] Nonetheless, there can be no doubt that harm is incurred when patients are diagnosed with a subclinical thyroid carcinoma that will never progress to clinical significance (overdiagnosis) or when children lose many quality years of life when the diagnosis is made too early.

Midorikawa and Ohtsuru observed the serious psychological, economic, and social harm of overdiagnosis (or diagnosis made too early) in the post-nuclear accident situation and became increasingly convinced of the need to revise the methodology of the thyroid examination. However, for most involved in the examination at that time, it was still difficult to comprehend the harms of overdiagnosis.

2. Struggle to reduce the harm of overdiagnosis (2015-2021)

1) Midorikawa and Ohtsuru's view on the overdiagnosis of thyroid cancer during the years 2015-2017

As many Japanese thyroid experts had speculated before the first round started, Midorikawa and Ohtsuru had also believed that most of the thyroid cancers detected in the first round would be early detection of clinically significant thyroid cancers (cancers that would become symptomatic a few years later). If this hypothesis is correct, the incidence of thyroid cancer would increase to some extent during the first round of screening but should return to a lower rate, the same as under a non-screening condition during the second round. To everyone's surprise, the rate of cancer detection in both the first and second rounds of screening was much higher than estimated from the above hypothesis, leading to the following questions. Were the unexpected numbers of cancers found in the first and second rounds of screening caused by radiation effect or the use of high-resolution imaging and liberal Japanese criteria for FNAC (nodules >5mm) or both? Were the majority of cancers being detected likely to become clinically significant or were they overdiagnosed?

In order to answer the question of whether the number of cancers detected in the first round of the thyroid examination was truly excessive, Takahashi et al.[15] developed a hypothetical simulation of expected cancer detection prevalence using an estimated high degree of US sensitivity, a median cancer sojourn period (length of time from the detectable incidental tumor to clinical detection) and data from the national cancer registry data. These authors concluded that the number of thyroid cancer cases detected in the first round was within the expected range based on a very high US sensitivity and a median sojourn times of 34 years (males) and 30 years (females) by the model as an exponential linear cell growth pattern. They also mentioned that the incidence of clinical thyroid cancer in children is low, favoring a long sojourn time, and they mentioned that the criteria for initiation of FNAC in the Japanese protocol could result in more detected cancers including detection of cancers that would never become clinically significant (overdiagnosis). Thus, given the use of high-resolution US screening and the liberal Japanese criteria for initiation of FNAC, Takahashi *et al.* did not consider the number of thyroid cancers detected in the first round of the thyroid examination excessive compared to what would be expected under non-accident conditions. They did mention the possibility of overdiagnosis, given the low cut-off criteria for FNAC in Japan.

However, this simulation does not account for the continued detection of thyroid cancers during the second round of screening. There are two theoretical explanations for this increased detection of thyroid cancer in the second and following rounds. The first is that the cancers are truly related to the radiation effect; however, this is highly unlikely given the very low estimated levels of radiation released following the accident, much lower than occurred in Chornobyl[16]. Mean thyroid equivalent doses of preschool children in Chornobyl were estimated to be 1548 mSv for evacuees and 449 mSv for residents of contaminated areas.[17] In contrast, the median thyroid equivalent doses of 1-year-old children range from 0.6 to 16 mSv in the evacuated area of Fukushima and far less in the remaining populated Fukushima.[18] No dose-dependent pattern emerged from the geographical distribution of absorbed doses by the municipality and the detection of thyroid cancer among participants within 4-6 years after the accident. Furthermore, radiation-induced thyroid cancer is well known to be more susceptible to radiation exposure at an early age. Thus, the distribution pattern of the number of thyroid cancers by the age of exposure should follow a pattern similar to Chornobyl, as shown in Fig. 7-1a.[19] The distribution pattern in Fukushima increased with older age and is not a pattern of radiation-induced thyroid cancer within five years in 2016 (Fig. 7-1b). Thyroid cancer will be detected even in the subjects who were younger at the time of the accident as chronological age increases. However, this age distribution pattern remained the same twelve years later, in 2023 (Fig. 7-1c).[20]

The second explanation is that many of these screen-detected cancers undergo growth arrest or regression and will never become clinically significant. This explanation had started to gain support by data showing a worldwide increase in US-detected thyroid cancers without significant changes in mortality and the active surveillance for papillary microcarcinomas (PMCs).

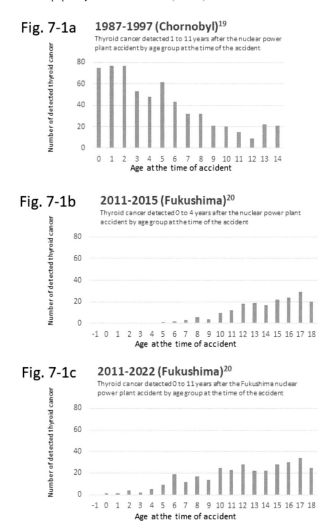

Fig 7-1 Comparison of thyroid cancer cases by age at the time of accident
(1a: Reprinted from reference 19 with permission from Springer Nature.
1b and 1c: Created by the author from publicly available data at the 50th meeting of the POCF.[20])

However, in 2015, the natural history of thyroid cancer prior to clinical cancer was not yet clear. So, we have tried to verify this hypothesis using US images from the primary and confirmatory examinations and revealed growth arrest pattern[21]. Reports from other research groups also provide evidence that most small papillary thyroid carcinomas (PTCs) undergo a period of proliferation followed by a slowing of growth, total growth arrest, or, in some cases, regression.[22, 23]

As discussed in Chapters 1 and 4, there is now data indicating that thyroid cancer develops in young people in an age-dependent fashion, with the majority becoming a US-detectable but asymptomatic in adolescence and young adulthood. The second round of the Fukushima thyroid examination was finding new US-detectable juvenile cancers in children who were 2-3 years older than during the first round (Fig.4-1). Ultimately, Midorikawa and Ohtsuru concluded that the design of the thyroid examination is likely to detect naturally occurring juvenile thyroid cancers, many or most of which would have remained asymptomatic for a lifetime if undetected by screening. Thus, overdiagnosis is occurring.

In addition to the problem of overdiagnosis, it has proven difficult to convince some people that the thyroid cancers detected via the thyroid examination are not related to radiation. The United Nations Scientific Committee on the Effects of Atomic Radiation (UNSCEAR) 2015 White Paper[16] had already noted that the radiation doses received by the residents of Fukushima were so low that an increased risk of thyroid cancer is unlikely. Additionally, studies of radiation epidemiology in areas affected by atomic bombings and nuclear experiments have shown that it is unlikely that thyroid cancer will increase owing to radiation exposure in the residents of Fukushima.[24] Children who have received computed tomography (CT) scans of the head and neck, lungs, or whole body due to illnesses or injuries have received higher doses of radiation than Fukushima residents. Given that CT scans have been widely used for diagnosis for over two decades, it is hard to imagine, based on scientific sense and previous studies, that the number of thyroid cancer cases would increase significantly at such low levels of radiation exposure.

2) Challenges to solve the problem of overdiagnosis (2015)

Midorikawa and Ohtsuru, have frequently shared their opinions on these matters at FMU. However, even experts in radiation medicine and thyroid diseases sometimes struggle to understand the concept of overdiagnosis and the new model of the natural history of thyroid cancer that explains it. Therefore, Midorikawa and Ohtsuru patiently continue to explain their views on the overdiagnosis issue. Eventually, Shinich Kikuchi, the President of FMU, and Masafumi Abe, the Executive Director of Radiation Medical Center, Koichi Tanigawa, the Vice-President of FMU came to recognize the problems caused by overdiagnosis.

They pointed out a problem with the thyroid examination administrative leadership. The person responsible for screening was also in charge of surgery. Thus, a conflict of interest might occur if surgical therapy was prioritized over addressing the harms of early detection and overtreatment. To avoid such conflicts of interest, the TUE was restructured in April 2015, with Ohtsuru as head and Midorikawa as vice head of the Department of Thyroid Ultrasound Examination. The president and the executive director believed that, although it was an extremely complex and challenging issue, reducing the harm of overdiagnosis could make the examination beneficial for the residents. Midorikawa and Ohtsuru accepted this responsibility and decided to do everything in their power for the patients and residents. However, in addition to their daily medical practice duties, they constantly had to address the concerns of a very large number of residents (referred to as the "silent majority") while caring for patients.

3) Attempt to modify the test methods to prevent overdiagnosis (2015-2017)

Midorikawa and Ohtsuru believed that overdiagnosis was occurring and that the number of thyroid cancers detected in the thyroid examination should be reduced. They found that the percentage of thyroid cancers between 5 mm and 10 mm detected in the second round was higher than in the first round. Therefore, they thought that increasing the cut-off screening value from >5 mm to >10 mm might reduce overdiagnosis by about a third. The American Thyroid Association issued guidelines in 2015 stating that FNAC is recommended for nodules ≥ 1cm and < 1.5 cm when they meet the US criteria for high or intermediate suspicion of malignancy with FNAC recommended for nodules ≥1.5 cm at lower levels of suspicion. Subcentimeter nodules may be followed without FNAC in the absence of evidence of extrathyroidal extension or cervical lymph node metastases.[25] This proposal to change the cut-off value was first presented to the Extramural Expert Committee, a subcommittee examining diagnostic criteria and is composed of prominent Japanese national thyroid specialists. The proposal to change the cut-off value in the third round received both supportive and opposing opinions and was ultimately brought to the Headquarters meeting. The Headquarters Meeting is attended by those responsible for the thyroid examination as well as various members involved in the FHMS. However, this proposal was not approved due to strong opposition from outside professors who are authorities in the field of radiation. They argued that changing the cut-off value would make the previous examination results meaningless and would not be socially acceptable.

The sizes of the nodules had already been recorded in previous examinations, so even if the cut-off value was changed, the data could still be compared to previous ones if the analysis was limited to nodules larger than 1cm. It was a question of finding a balance between reducing overdiagnosis and maintaining the protocol of the examination as written in order to ensure consistency. The decision suggests that priority was given to ensuring protocol consistency and failed to address the need to assess and modify the screening program in order to reduce potential harm. Since the plan was rejected at the Headquarters Meeting, it became impossible to change the examination method. As a result, an opportunity to mitigate the harm of overdiagnosis was missed.

In November 2016, Abe, the Executive Director of Radiation Medical Center, who understood the need to reform the thyroid examination to reduce the harm of overdiagnosis, was transferred. In this challenging situation, Midorikawa and Ohtsuru tried to make some partial improvements. For example, they added a new checkbox to the consent form for the third round to allow subjects to indicate not only their consent but also their non-consent. They also added a statement to the notification letter sent to the subjects that "a thyroid US examination is not generally recommended for asymptomatic people and may cause anxiety rather than a relief," although they were not allowed to explain overdiagnosis in detail. In other words, FMU and Fukushima Prefecture were not proactive in communicating about overdiagnosis to the residents. As a result, it was not possible to establish a system to help the subjects and their caregivers make informed decisions about whether to undergo thyroid examinations and be aware of the potential harm of overdiagnosis.

In 2016, the fifth memorial year of the nuclear power plant accident was marked by several international conferences. At these international conferences, Midorikawa and Ohtsuru gave presentations on the topic of thyroid examination with the following remarks [4, 26]

1. The thyroid examination is causing the harm of overdiagnosis
2. The examination creates a significant psychosocial burden, such as anxiety
3. Obtaining consent based on explaining the harm of the examination, including overdiagnosis, is necessary.
4. Participation in the examination should be voluntary

Prior to these conferences, some domestic researchers had also recognized the issue of overdiagnosis in the Fukushima thyroid examination.[10, 27] However, this perspective was not widely known. Midorikawa and Ohtsuru's presentations brought greater awareness of the problem of overdiagnosis and the need for change in the thyroid examination process in Fukushima. On the other hand, some experts became very nervous about using the term "overdiagnosis." For instance, there was confusion over the terminology within the Extramural Expert Committee, as some experts interpreted "overdiagnosis" as "misdiagnosis." At an international conference, a doctor requested that the term "overdiagnosis" not be used in the context of Fukushima, stating that it was hurtful.

Initially, most experts within FMU were not particularly concerned about the increasing number of thyroid cancers. However, in late 2016 and early 2017, FMU was frequently asked for its opinion on overdiagnosis. As a result, FMU needed to reach a consensus on its stance. To gather opinions within FMU, Tanigawa, the Vice President of FMU organized a consensus meeting on the thyroid examination. During the meeting, it was agreed that the current thyroid examination method may result in many overdiagnosed cases; however, no decision was made to modify its method. It was concluded that many people seem to undergo the examination without knowing the major disadvantages, including overdiagnosis, and that a survey was necessary to determine how the subjects and their caregivers perceive the thyroid examination. This survey could be done through questionnaires. Additionally, it was proposed that an analysis be done to examine the relationship between school examinations and the screening participation rate.

Midorikawa and Ohtsuru began these projects immediately. However, FMU responded in an inexplicable manner. A questionnaire survey was planned and discussed at several related meetings. Just as the research was about to begin, FMU suddenly withdrew funding for the research, and the survey was delayed for years. Midorikawa and Ohtsuru also wrote a paper analyzing the relationship between school examinations and the participation rate, suggesting that the examinations conducted at schools may have increased the participation rate, but they may not have ensured that participation was voluntary. However, the review committee at FMU, which is responsible for granting permission to the researchers to submit papers using data from the FHMS, refused to issue permission for this paper submission.

Thus, even though there were some meeting attendees who favored addressing the problem of overdiagnosis, FMU used various tactics to effectively prohibit the implementation of research that could hinder the continuation of the thyroid examination, even if such research could provide beneficial information to the residents.

This policy prevents the residents of Fukushima from understanding the reality and significance of the thyroid examination and the harm of overdiagnosis. It may also distort the perceptions of researchers who receive scientific information from FMU.

In late 2016, the Ministry of the Environment proposed that Fukushima Prefecture receive a comprehensive review and recommendations from an international organization as an independent third party on thyroid cancer screening after the nuclear accident. The 2018 International Agency for Research on Cancer (IARC) Expert Group on Thyroid Health Monitoring after Nuclear Accidents (TM-NUC) reviewed the activities following nuclear accidents in Fukushima and other locations. In conclusion, the IARC Expert Group "recommends against population thyroid screening after a nuclear accident."[28, 29] IARC also states, "The guiding principle for any health intervention should be to maximize benefit and minimize harm, and this approach should also be considered with respect to thyroid health monitoring."[29]

4) Forces against efforts to curb overdiagnosis (2017-2021)

The following describes the status of related academic societies in Japan. The Japan Thyroid Association (JTA) and the Japan Association of Endocrine Surgery (JAES), along with other US-related associations, have provided various support for the Fukushima thyroid examination since its inception. This includes providing personnel for ultrasonography and conducting examinations for subjects who have moved to other prefectures. Additionally, the JTA has identified "thyroid US examination in the FHMS" as an issue of clinical importance, and as of April 2021, sixteen members including some professors from FMU were on the JTA experts committee. However, its activities are largely unpublished, and no written statements from this committee regarding the relationship between thyroid cancer and radiation exposure or overdiagnosis have been made public. The head of the committee has occasionally commented at annual meetings of the JTA, stating that measures are already in place to prevent overdiagnosis and minimize the harm. In essence, the discussion of overdiagnosis has long been taboo within the JTA, and there has been no discussion of this problem within society.

At the annual meeting of the Japan Endocrine Society in April 2017, Ohtsuru pointed out potential overdiagnosis in the Fukushima thyroid examination at a symposium on thyroid cancer screening. Midorikawa also reported on the psychosocial impact of thyroid examinations and the harm of thyroid cancer screening at a symposium on the Fukushima nuclear accident organized by the Council for Gender Equality. The audience gained some understanding of these issues, and Midorikawa and Ohtsuru hoped that this would be the start of a discussion leading to a reevaluation of the TUE process in Fukushima. However, an anti-nuclear power group sent a letter of inquiry to the president of FMU regarding the report at this congress, stating that the issue of overdiagnosis could reduce the participation rate and risk delaying diagnosis. This letter led to another taboo against mentioning overdiagnosis at FMU. Henceforth, overdiagnosis of thyroid cancer was not presented as a major topic of discussion in the Japan Endocrine Society.

In Japan, where thyroid cancer screening is conducted, there are two likely reasons for the lack of discussion on the issue of overdiagnosis. First, the belief that thyroid cancers are caused by radiation exposure after a nuclear accident is fundamental to the operations of the anti-nuclear movement. Anti-nuclear groups are reluctant to accept that many thyroid cancers occur in the absence of radiation exposure or that both radiation-associated and spontaneous thyroid cancers are, for the most part, self-limiting or indolent papillary carcinomas. The second reason is a reluctance to criticize the thyroid examination owing to a desire to show respect for the experts involved in thyroid screening as part of post-nuclear health checkups in both Fukushima and Chornobyl.

Kikuchi retired as the President of FMU in March 2017. From mid-2017 onwards, FMU discouraged Midorikawa and Ohtsuru from explaining overdiagnosis and its harms. Also, they were not allowed to express opinions on the ethics of the school examinations and whether the program is truly voluntary. Permission was not granted for an explanation of overdiagnosis and potential harms to be included in the explanatory meeting handouts for the residents and attendees in classes on the school-based TUE. The shelving of the survey questionnaires and suspension of the submission of questionnaire-related manuscripts also occurred around the same time.

Thyroid examinations are conducted at hospitals and facilities in prefectures other than Fukushima for subjects who have moved elsewhere in Japan. From FY2016 to FY2017, FMU conducted a project commissioned by the Ministry of the Environment and the Nuclear Safety Research Association of Japan to provide explanations and information to collaborators involved in the examinations outside of Fukushima. The Ministry of the Environment requested that FMU participants minimize the discussion of the harm of overdiagnosis in the thyroid examination when providing explanations and information. Midorikawa and Ohtsuru refused to do so because they believe that sharing information on overdiagnosis is one of the most important aspects of this project. As a result, they were subsequently removed from the project.

Since 2014, there has been almost no discussion on overdiagnosis at the POCF and TFTE meetings, and there has been a tendency to avoid any related discussions. For example, in 2016, the Fukushima Pediatric Association requested a review of the thyroid examination in Fukushima Prefecture, but the POCF did not accept this request as a topic for discussion. Recommendations on the TUE compiled at the aforementioned international symposium in 2016 were submitted to Fukushima Prefecture, stating that it is essential to ensure that participation in the examination is completely voluntary. However, this, too, was not discussed at the POCF and TFTE meetings.

The POCF and TFTE members serve two-year terms, and some new members were elected in 2017. These committee members are nominated by professional societies and other organizations and appointed by Fukushima Prefecture. At a meeting, some new committee members raised the issue of overdiagnosis, accountability for harm related to the examination, and ethical issues such as semi-compulsory participation in school examinations. At the 10th and 11th meetings of the TFTE in 2018, the recommendations made by Tomotaka Sobue and Toru Takano (Osaka University) were discussed (Table 4-2). In this proposal, the inadequacies and problems with the instructions for the TUE were pointed out, and a suggestion for their revision was also presented.[30, 31] The discussion at the meetings was turbulent, and in the end, the chairperson of the TFTE handled these recommendations. Only problems concerning the explanatory document were discussed. At these meetings, FMU proposed a new explanatory document that is currently in use. The document does not include the term "overdiagnosis," and the recommendations by Sobue and Takano have only partially been implemented.

After these discussions, Fukushima Prefecture assigned the TFTE the role of conducting analyses related to thyroid cancer and radiation exposure and prohibited the discussion of other matters. For example, at the TFTE meeting in 2021, the UNSCEAR 2020 report was introduced, stating that the radiation dose in Fukushima was so low that thyroid cancer would not be expected to increase and that the unexpected number of thyroid cancers detected may be due to overdiagnosis caused by sensitive US examination.[32] However, in response to the opinion that this information should be made known to examination subjects and other residents, the chairman stated that this was not something to be discussed in the TFTE.

In the POCF, problems with school examinations were sometimes discussed. However, concerns about the seemingly compulsory nature of school screening and subjects not being sufficiently aware of the risks of the examination were offset by the argument that examinations at school are more convenient for those who are anxious. Thus, these concerns were never discussed intensively. It appears that the focus of the thyroid examination had become acquiring data on the health effects of radiation rather than monitoring children's health. From an ethical point of view, the goal of the thyroid examination should be clearly stated in the consent form, including that participants themselves may not benefit from the survey and that harm may occur. It was desirable to discuss concrete plans for how to prevent ethical problems from arising. However, Fukushima Prefecture and FMU did not deepen the discussion, saying the ethics committee of FMU had examined the ethical issues and approved the thyroid examination as no problem.

Around this time, many experts in various fields pointed out the problem of overdiagnosis in the thyroid examination in magazines and social networking sites. However, at the end of March 2018, while these discussions were still taking place, Midorikawa and Ohtsuru were asked to resign from their responsibilities for the TUE.

Section 3
What does the thyroid examination mean to each person involved?

1. Children do not want their caregivers to be sad

School examinations are performed during school hours, and there is not enough time for the medical staff to talk with each child individually. One school requested that FMU offer explanatory meetings for groups of parents with the children. In 2014, Midorikawa began offering classes on the TUE to children.

She knew that many children were anxious about the examination, concerned about the result, and had the mistaken belief that the examination measures the degree of radiation exposure. At the beginning of the class, she used to say, "Do you know where your thyroid gland is? Please touch where your thyroid gland is." Almost all the children touched the correct location of their thyroid glands. Adults probably could not do this. Information regarding the thyroid gland's location and biology is not generally taught to the general public. The children in Fukushima have undergone thyroid examinations, so they know the location of the thyroid gland from experience. Next, she asked, "Do you know why you have thyroid examinations?" Although a few students answered with the word "radiation," most did not know why they underwent thyroid examinations.[4] This became more apparent each time the classes were given, leading Midorikawa to realize that explanations about the examination still needed to be provided.

In the early days, the content of the classes included topics such as why the thyroid examination is being conducted, what is the function of the thyroid gland and iodine, the level of radioactive iodine is lower than those in Chornobyl, what can we learn from a US examination, cysts are nothing to worry about, and the examination will continue for a long time. Thyroid cancer was missing from these topics of discussion. However, as more cases of cancer were detected, Midorikawa began to explain that most nodules are considered benign and that even thyroid cancer is often highly curable. There was some resistance within FMU to explaining overdiagnosis, but she began to emphasize that some thyroid cancers may remain asymptomatic throughout a person's lifetime.

The children were asked to write down their impressions after the class. Midorikawa learned a great deal from their writings. Many of them stated that they were relieved to know that cysts are not a concern and that their mothers would be happy to hear this. As mentioned earlier, cysts (category A2) worried many mothers (see Chapter 3). It was clear that the children were also concerned and did not want their mothers to worry. Additionally, many of them said they were glad to know why they underwent the thyroid examination. Some said they were glad or proud to know that Fukushima was safe based on the examination results, even though they understood that radiation exposure was low enough not to cause illness. However, there were also occasional descriptions of anxiety, such as "What will happen the next time a nuclear power plant explodes?" and "Will we continue to be discriminated against?" The children had not been informed that the examination could harm them, nor did they know that the examination cannot determine whether Fukushima is safe or not. Upon reading these responses, Midorikawa felt sorry and strongly regretted allowing children to feel this anxiety and be deprived of more complete explanations.

It seems that many parents wanted their children to undergo thyroid examinations out of a sense of obligation and a desire to be reassured that they had not exposed their children to radiation. Some even wanted their children examined in order to prove that they were healthy and allow them to eventually marry. The children understand that their parents care about them and act to spare their parents' feelings. This is especially true in the case of cysts and when they are diagnosed with nodules or thyroid cancer. One patient who was diagnosed with thyroid cancer in the FHMS recounted that he had undergone a thyroidectomy to spare his mother's feelings. Upon hearing this, Midorikawa thought that if the thyroid examination had been improved and overdiagnosis had been suppressed sooner, it might have been possible to prevent anyone from having such an irrational experience.

2. Emotional conflict among medical staff involved in the thyroid examination

Many medical staff and officers are involved in the thyroid examination. While physicians perform specialist tasks such as FNAC and data analysis, clinical technologists are primarily responsible for performing US thyroid cancer screening, and clerks manage data and prepare documents. Many of these people are residents of Fukushima, are related to the subjects, believe that the thyroid examination is beneficial to the residents, and mean well when they perform the examinations. They are dedicated to this work, even if it is sometimes painful for them. The sadness and stress they feel when the residents, anxious about the examination result, complain about them must be significant. Additionally, they may find it unreasonable to have the disadvantages of the thyroid examination, such as overdiagnosis, pointed out because they are involved in the screening as part of their work for the university.

The more mindful medical staff and administrative officers are, the more significant the conflict over the thyroid examination becomes. It is difficult for them to think their hard work may not benefit others. However, this "awareness" should begin with understanding the residents' situation. The TUE examinees may incur harm without the benefit of having received a complete explanation of the TUE's risks. The following is a record of the struggles experienced by a clinical technologist who was involved in the TUE during the early days but has now left the scene.

"Experience as an ultrasonographer in thyroid examination"
Manabu Ohishi

When we became staff members involved in thyroid examinations, our supervisors and physicians told us that this was a highly focused project of great social importance. Especially in the early days of the thyroid examination, each of us had a strong sense of mission to work for "reconstruction" and "resolving the concerns of the prefectural residents." Staff from various professions were brought from within and outside the prefecture, and we felt that the work being done here would surely benefit society someday. The thyroid examination required direct communication with the residents of Fukushima Prefecture, as children were the examination subjects. Few national or prefectural government projects conducted at FMU directly involved the residents. Therefore, we recognized that this was a vital work site where we needed to listen to the voices of the prefectural residents, including their complaints and concerns. After a while, I began to wonder if there was anything we could do to give back to the children and their parents beyond just performing the ultrasound examinations. For example, I wanted to help them understand the examination as much as possible and alleviate their anxiety. Everything was new to us; we were learning as we went along, but I was happy when

I heard the voice of the prefectural residents.

When the second round of examination started, I saw many children become anxious as they remembered the previous first round. Children's anxiety is not limited to examination results. Some children felt anxious and burdened by the examination itself. The fact that the examination results were not good or that there were findings contrary to expectations left a bad impression on the children about thyroid examinations. This "something" is not just cancer. Even benign tumors and cysts found in many people caused anxiety. Once I understood the problem of overdiagnosis, I became very doubtful about detecting thyroid cancer as I saw anxious children. As ultrasonographers who go out to the examination venue as medical technologists, we will find thyroid tumors at a specific rate. If we examine 100-200 children, we find thyroid tumors. We routinely perform hundreds of examinations each week. Most of what we detected in this way are benign tumors and nothing to worry about, but some are thyroid cancers found in one out of several thousand children. I was concerned about whether I was doing the right thing as a medical technologist. The impact on a young person's life for decades to come, both for the child and their parents, is immeasurable if they are diagnosed with thyroid cancer. For example, a child who was joking around with friends and enjoying studies and club activities yesterday would suddenly face despair if they knew they have thyroid cancer. Contrary to what my boss initially told me, I became increasingly uncertain whether the thyroid examination was really for the benefit of the Fukushima residents and children. I feel so strongly about this because statistical data and evidence show that few people die from thyroid cancer. Given the general belief that cancer must be detected and treated early, it seemed strange. However, many people are diagnosed with thyroid cancer and live without symptoms for decades without treatment. Knowing these facts, I began to wonder if it is a proper medical practice to diagnose teenagers with thyroid cancer.

However, as mentioned above, the thyroid examination is a highly focused and socially significant project, a political cover. It seems as if the thyroid examination was not allowed to stop, with huge funds being invested in the project by the national and prefectural governments. It was like a steam locomotive without brakes being fed endless fuel. At some point, I became horrified at the prospect of the thyroid examination as a running business. Moreover, even though it is a project funded with public money, it seems to be detrimental to the children. Children are almost automatically put through a system of thyroid examinations. In this system, they are only told how to take the examination, and in the worst-case scenario, they are told,

"You have thyroid cancer," without being fully informed about the examination. In many cases, children who are told they have cancer are put on a separate system to undergo surgery. Some children regret having taken the examination without knowing anything about it. It is not surprising that a cancer diagnosis can provoke fear of death in some children. I began to think that perhaps thyroid examinations that lead to overdiagnosis are "fear sentences" for children.

Who should determine the necessity of continued thyroid examinations? It should be the children subjected to the thyroid examination, not those who promote them. More than ten years have passed since the disaster, and I believe the children are now old enough to make their own decisions. It is necessary to ask the children again. We should ask the children whether they want to take a thyroid examination. This choice should be made after thoroughly discussing the fact that the risk of thyroid cancer is unlikely to increase with the radiation dose in Fukushima, the possibility of overdiagnosing thyroid cancer, and the harm it can cause.

3. **Problems with media coverage in Fukushima**

Early media reports on the thyroid examination in Fukushima Prefecture were characterized by accusations that FMU was not providing sufficient information and was evading responsibility. As thyroid cancer cases began to be detected, media reports changed to focus on the number of people with thyroid cancer in Fukushima. When the POCF and others suggested that there was a low likelihood of a causal relationship with radiation exposure, some media outlets questioned or criticized these reports. The presence of certain media outlets reporting with a biased belief that there must be health effects from radiation exposure often drowned out voices from other outlets reporting that "Fukushima is fine." Although there was limited reporting on the low risk of radiation, it was treated as a minor issue. As a result, the media gave little attention to the possibility of overdiagnosis in Fukushima's thyroid examination. Reporting on overdiagnosis is often viewed as a false or misleading report that downplays or denies the effects of radiation exposure.

Scientifically, overdiagnosis and radiation effects are two distinct issues. US screening can result in overdiagnosis of thyroid cancer regardless of whether tumors are spontaneous or radiation-associated. To evaluate the effects of radiation and concomitantly minimize overdiagnosis, one should consider the use of a national registry of thyroid cancer cases reported based on clinical diagnoses rather than screening. As suggested by IARC, such registries can be used to characterize the geographical variation of tumor incidence and prevalence following a nuclear accident or other event resulting in the release of toxic materials.[29] It would also be more effective to address individuals' anxieties personally rather than offering a one-size-fits-all screening approach. Some journalists who understood this began to report scientifically on overdiagnosis and the low risk of radiation-induced cancer to the affected people, while some media outlets continued to present thyroid cancer in Fukushima as a health hazard caused by radiation.

Many media outlets seem to be presenting both sides of the argument about radiation and thyroid cancer simultaneously in a general manner that can cause confusion and misinterpretation of risks. In science, there is no such thing as 0% or 100% certainty. It is essential to carefully explain that uncertainty is always present in medicine; however, science-based estimates of probability should be clearly communicated to the public. When there are disputes between opposing groups, there must be a mechanism to convey to the public that risk estimates are based on scientific evidence and not motivated by personal or political agendas. For example, there is scientific consensus that the probability of an increase in thyroid cancer due to radiation exposure in Fukushima is very low, close to 0%. This must be carefully explained to the public with supportive data so that the residents do not interpret the situation as "the effects of radiation are unknown. As the risk is not zero." Such communications are always difficult because of the human tendency to favor one side of any argument via affect heuristics rather than statistical data.[33]

Ochi argues that experts dealing with nuclear accidents or other types of disasters that release invisible hazards must carefully explain the science while considering differences in individuals' beliefs and cultures. Also, these experts must understand that post-disaster experiences, emotions, personal values, and ideology can influence decision-making more than statistics and science.[34] Thus, one needs to explain that the probability of radiation causing thyroid cancer in Fukushima is extremely low based on scientific analyses. However, experts must try to understand and respect the views of residents and refrain from criticizing those who choose to undergo thyroid screening owing to fear of radiation-induced cancer. The same care must be taken when discussing the harms of screening and overdiagnosis. Experts need to recognize that the explanation of overdiagnosis can lead patients to feel blamed for being screened.

On the other hand, experts should not refrain from discussing overdiagnosis with anxious patients because overdiagnosis and diagnosis too early can lead to patient suffering. Discussions, however, should be done with respect and sympathy for patients' fears. The aim of shared decision-making after disaster should be, as discussed by Ochi, to develop mutual trust between residents and experts.[34] With mutual trust comes the opportunity to mitigate the adverse effects of media-generated misinformation and confusion.

4. Difficulty in modifying the thyroid examination by personnel affiliated with FMU

Midorikawa and Ohtsuru assumed responsibility for the operation of the TUE in the middle of the second round in 2015. They implemented the efforts previously described in order to improve its inadequacies as a "watching for the health of the residents," reduce anxiety caused by the examination, and reduce overdiagnosis as much as possible. Since around 2017, these efforts have faced increasing restraint by FMU, Fukushima Prefecture, and in some cases, the Ministry of the Environment.

Fukushima Prefecture commissioned FMU to plan and conduct the thyroid examination and distributed the budget. However, this led to a strange situation where it was deemed inappropriate for someone within FMU to evaluate the examination or to point out any problems because FMU was not considered to have the authority to make decisions about whether to conduct the examination. If it is impossible to address an issue that is causing harmful effects, this system is problematic. The current thyroid screening method was not devised or directed by Fukushima Prefecture but was solely orchestrated by FMU. The thyroid examination was proposed to the prefecture before the harms of screening were widely known and before publications of recommendations against population screening for thyroid cancer. Thus, one can understand why there were flaws in the program design, but why not implement changes designed to minimize harms?

Midorikawa and Ohtsuru continued to conduct the third round of the examination (2016-2018) in much the same way, with some workplace modifications and changes in how results were released, as described previously. Despite various forms of resistance, they were able to publish several science-based manuscripts related to overdiagnosis and its potential harms.[35-37] In addition, there have been publications aimed at education of the endocrinologists and cytopathologists. Midorikawa and Ohtsuru have authored a chapter in an English-language textbook, *Thyroid FNA Cytology (Springer)* aimed at informing specialists about considerations that should be given prior to thyroid FNA on children.[38] Here are some contents of the chapter. Prior to the performance of FNAC on asymptomatic children or young adults, there is a need for shared decision-making and informed consent for them. Consideration should be given to the fear and guilt that may accompany US and FNAC reports. Written reports of both benign and "malignant" lesions may generate negative feelings in both patients and caregivers when given without face-to-face explanations of the meanings of these reports. Patients and caretakers must fully understand the significance of these diagnoses and be allowed to ask questions.

Based on the guiding principle that all healthcare interventions should be designed to maximize benefit and minimize harm, it is unfortunate that certain ethical issues were not addressed prior to initiation of the thyroid examination. Participation in the thyroid examination should be purely voluntary; include healthcare literacy training with complete informed consent stating potential risks and benefits; and there should be face-to-face dialogues with participants to minimize anxiety. As part of informed consent, there should have been an acknowledgement that, to date, there is no evidence to suggest that the survey will provide health benefits to participants, and the only benefit may be the acquisition of research data to increase general knowledge about thyroid cancer epidemiology.

While actively conducting the second and third survey rounds, Midorikawa and Ohtsuru repeatedly discussed and proposed TUE changes designed to minimize harm to subjects. These included the need to provide a more complete and improved consent form and to improve explanatory material for the residents. They had hoped to improve the situation by the fourth or, at the latest, the fifth round of the thyroid examination. However, as mentioned previously, both left their TUE positions in 2018 before reaching their goals. In 2018, they assumed responsibility for the Office of Health Communication, which handles communication with residents related to the FHMS. As such, they initiated efforts to provide explanations of overdiagnosis at public facilities before thyroid examinations. They found that even into the third round, most examinees still knew nothing about overdiagnosis.

In contrast to the policy of FMU and Fukushima Prefecture to continue the thyroid examination, Nuclear Emergency Situation-Improvement of Medical and Health Surveillance (SHAMISEN) in late 2017 and IARC in 2018 reported that population screening for thyroid cancer is not recommended after a nuclear accident.[28, 39, 40] Reasons given for this recommendation were that the harms, including overdiagnosis, likely outweighed the benefits. UNSCEAR reassessed Fukushima radiation risks in their Sources, Effects and Risks of Ionizing Radiation 2020/2021 report and concluded that radiation exposure doses in Fukushima were too low to pose increased risk of childhood thyroid cancer.[32] Section 250 of Annex B (p97) states, "Care is needed in interpreting the results from sensitive ultrasound thyroid screening following radiation exposure after a major radiological accident. There is compelling evidence that sensitive ultrasound screening detects many more cases of thyroid cancer than would be detected following the presentation of clinical symptoms. The consequential over-diagnosis of thyroid cancer has the potential to cause anxiety among those screened and might lead to unnecessary treatment."

By this time, the opinions published by overseas experts had some influence on members of the POCF. Some members pointed out the issue of overdiagnosis and argued that the examination should be reviewed. Additionally, some former members of the POCF who had previously supported continuing the thyroid examination later stated that school examinations should at least be eliminated.

However, from 2018 to 2019, Midorikawa and Ohtsuru had increasing restrictions forced on their work related to overdiagnosis. The Vice-President of FMU, who was well aware of the problem of overdiagnosis, was also transferred in March 2019. FMU prohibited Midorikawa and Ohtsuru from presenting their views at international conferences, and the people who had supported them at FMU resigned one after another. The department to which they belonged was eventually in danger of being dissolved. They could no longer provide medical care, educate students about the problems of overdiagnosis, or conduct research to address these issues. They decided to resign from FMU in March 2020. Some of their colleagues remained at FMU and are still working hard to address many medical and health issues in Fukushima Prefecture. Of course, there are others who feel the same way as Midorikawa and Ohtsuru about the thyroid examination. However, the problems of the thyroid examination cannot be solved from the bottom up. FMU leadership needs to assume a major role in the redesign and implementation of a policy-making of the thyroid examination.

The problem of thyroid cancer overdiagnosis and overtreatment of thyroid nodules in general has become globally recognized. Awareness of this problem should be a call for dispassionate debate and discussion of evidence-based data with the intent to promote the well-being of patients and "do no harm." Neutral third-party, science-based evidence should be welcomed even when it may not be what one wants to hear. As a center of learning, a university should strive to welcome input from scientists on both sides of a controversy, domestic and international, and give regard to recommendations from international expert groups.

The people of Fukushima have gradually overcome the Great East Japan Earthquake and the nuclear power plant accident, even though they are victims of the disaster. Midorikawa, Ohtsuru, and many of their colleagues have endeavored to reduce the harms of the thyroid examination by offering their expertise to educate, comfort, and reduce stress and anxiety. They hope to continue to provide as much support as possible to the young people of Fukushima and their caretakers.

References

1. Suzuki S, et al, The protocol and preliminary baseline survey results of the thyroid ultrasound examination in Fukushima. *Endocr J* 63: 315-21, 2016.
2. Yasumura S, et al. Study protocol for the Fukushima Health Management Survey. *J Epidemiol* 22:375-83, 2012.
3. Hino Y, et al. Explanatory meetings on thyroid examination for the "Fukushima Health Management Survey" after the Great East Japan Earthquake: Reduction of anxiety and improvement of comprehension. *Tohoku J Exper Medicine* 239: 333-43, 2016.
4. Midorikawa S, et al. Psychosocial issues related to thyroid examination after a radiation disaster. *Asia Pac J Pub Health* 29: 63S-73S, 2017.
5. Midorikawa S, et al. Psychosocial impact of the thyroid examination of the Fukushima Health Management Survey. In: Thyroid cancer and nuclear accidents: Long-term aftereffects of Chernobyl and Fukushima (1st ed.). Academic Press, pp.165-73, 2017.
6. Tsugane S, Radiation exposure and thyroid cancer after the Fukushima nuclear accident : the effect of overdiagnosis in causal relationship assessment. *J Jpn Thyroid Assoc* 12:45-51, 2021 (in Japanese).
7. Hasegawa A. Initial turmoil in an emergency situation. In: Heath Effects of the Fukushima Nuclear Disaster. Academic Press, pp.23-40, 2022.
8. Japan Consortium of Juvenile Thyroid Cancer. Japan: Midorikawa S.: Will of Dr. Nagataki. [internet, cited 2024 July 15] Available from: https://jcjtc.org/en/essay/61/.
9. Fukushima Prefecture. Fukushima, Japan: Minutes of the 2nd meeting of the Task Force for Thyroid Examination (in Japanese). [internet, cited 2024 July 15] Available from: https://www.pref.fukushima.lg.jp/uploaded/attachment/62600.pdf.
10. Shibuya K, et al. Time to reconsider thyroid cancer screening in Fukushima. *Lancet* 383: 1883-4, 2014.
11. Fukushima Prefecture. Fukushima, Japan: Meeting material submitted by Yoshikazu Nishi at the 2nd meeting of the Task Force for Thyroid Examination (in Japanese). [internet, cited 2024 July 15] Available from: https://www.pref.fukushima.lg.jp/uploaded/attachment/50321.pdf.
12. Fukushima Prefecture. Fukushima, Japan: Comments on the evaluation of the results of the thyroid examination in the Fukushima Health Management Survey (in Japanese). [internet, cited 2024 July 15] Available from: https://www.pref.fukushima.lg.jp/uploaded/attachment/50322.pdf.
13. Ahn HS, et al. Korea's thyroid-cancer "epidemic"--screening and overdiagnosis. *N*

Engl J Med 371: 1765-7, 2014.
14. Hofmann B, *et al*. Overdiagnosis, one concept, three perspectives, and a model. *Eur J Epidemiol* 36:361-6, 2021.
15. Takahashi H, *et al.* Simulation of expected childhood and adolescent thyroid cancer cases in Japan using a cancer-progression model based on the National Cancer Registry: application to the first-round thyroid examination of the Fukushima Health Management Survey. *Medicine (Baltimore)* 96: e8631, 2017.
16. United Nations Scientific Committee on the Effects of Atomic Radiation. Vienna, Austria: Developments since the 2013 UNSCEAR report of the levels and effects of radiation exposure due to the nuclear accident following the Great East-Japan earthquake and tsunami. A 2015 White Paper to guide the Scientific Committee's future programme of work. [internet, cited 2024 July 15] Available from: https://www.unscear.org/unscear/uploads/documents/publications/UNSCEAR_2015 _WP.pdf.
17. United Nations Scientific Committee on the Effects of Atomic Radiation. Vienna, Austria: UNSCEAR 2008 report volume I. Sources of ionizing radiation. Available from: https://www.unscear.org/unscear/en/publications/2008_1.html.
18. Ohba T, *et al.* Reconstruction of residents' thyroid equivalent doses from internal radionuclides after the Fukushima Daiichi nuclear power station accident. *Sci Rep* 10:3639, 2020.
19. Williams D. Radiation carcinogenesis: lessons from Chernobyl. *Oncogene* 27 S9-18, 2009.
20. Fukushima Prefecture. Fukushima, Japan: Materials from the 50th meeting of the Prefectural Oversight Committee for the FHMS (in Japanese). [internet, cited 2024 July 15] Available from: https://www.pref.fukushima.lg.jp/sec/21045b/kenkocyosa-kentoiinkai-50.html.
21. Midorikawa S, *et al.* Comparative analysis of the growth pattern of thyroid cancer in young patients screened by ultrasonography in Japan after a nuclear accident: The Fukushima Health Management Survey. *JAMA Otolaryngol Head Neck Surg* 144:57–63, 2018.
22. Ito Y, *et al.* Kinetic analysis of growth activity in enlarging papillary microcarcinomas. *Thyroid* 29:1765-73, 2019.
23. Tuttle RM, *et al.* Active surveillance of papillary thyroid carcinoma: frequency and time course of the six most common tumor volume kinetic patterns. *Thyroid* 32:1337-45, 2022.
24. Nagataki S, *et al.* Measurements of individual radiation doses in residents living

around the Fukushima Nuclear Power Plant. *Radiat Res* 180:439-47, 2013.
25. Haugen BR, et al. 2015 American Thyroid Association management guidelines for adult patients with thyroid nodules and differentiated thyroid cancer. *Thyroid* 26: 1-133, 2016.
26. Ohtsuru A, et al. Five-year interim report of thyroid ultrasound examinations in the Fukushima Health Management Survey. In: Thyroid cancer and nuclear accidents: Long-term after effects of Chernobyl and Fukushima (1st ed.). Academic Press, pp.145-53, 2017.
27. Katanoda K, et al. Quantification of the increase in thyroid cancer prevalence in Fukushima after the nuclear disaster in 2011--a potential overdiagnosis? *Jpn J Clin Oncol* 46: 284-6, 2016.
28. Togawa K, et al. Long-term strategies for thyroid health monitoring after nuclear accidents: recommendations from an Expert Group convened by IARC. *Lancet Oncol* 19: 1280-3, 2018.
29. International Agency for Research on Cancer. Lyon, France: Thyroid health monitoring after nuclear accidents. IARC technical publication No.46. [internet, cited 2024 July 15] Available from: https://publications.iarc.fr/Book-And-Report-Series/Iarc-Technical-Publications/Thyroid-Health-Monitoring-After-Nuclear-Accidents-2018.
30. Fukushima Prefecture. Fukushima, Japan: Ethical issues and improvement proposals for the thyroid ultrasound examination in Fukushima Health Management Survey (in Japanese). [internet, cited 2024 July 15] Available from: https://www.pref.fukushima.lg.jp/uploaded/attachment/278764.pdf.
31. Fukushima Prefecture. Fukushima, Japan: Problems and improvement proposals for the implementation system and method of the thyroid ultrasound examination in the Fukushima Health Management Survey (in Japanese). [internet, cited 2024 July 15] Available from: https://www.pref.fukushima.lg.jp/uploaded/attachment/295104.pdf.
32. United Nations Scientific Committee on the Effects of Atomic Radiation. Viena, Austria: Sources, Effects and Risks of Ionizing Radiation 2020/2021 Report. Volume II, Scientific Annex B. [internet, cited 2024 July 15] Available from: https://www.unscear.org/unscear/uploads/documents/unscear-reports/UNSCEAR_2020_21_Report_Vol.II.pdf.
33. Slovic P, et al. Affect, risk and decision making. *Health Psychol* 24:S35-40, 2005.
34. Ochi S. 'Life communication' after the 2011 Fukushima nuclear disaster: what experts need to learn from residential non-scientific rationality. *J Radiat Res* 62:i88-i94, 2021.

35. Ohtsuru A, et al. Incidence of thyroid cancer among children and young adults in Fukushima, Japan, screened with 2 rounds of ultrasonography within 5 years of the 2011 Fukushima Daiichi Nuclear Power Station accident. *JAMA Otolaryngol Head Neck Surg* 145:4–11, 2019.
36. Midorikawa S, et al. Harm of overdiagnosis or extremely early diagnosis behind trends in pediatric thyroid cancer. *Cancer* 125:4108-9, 2019.
37. Midorikawa S, et al. Disaster-zone research: make participation voluntary. *Nature* 579:193, 2020.
38. Midorikawa S, Ohtsuru A. How to be considerate to patients with thyroid nodules: lessons from the pediatric thyroid cancer center screening program in Fukushima after the nuclear plant accident. In: Thyroid FNA and cytology: Differential diagnosis and pitfalls. Springer, pp.95-9, 2019.
39. Institut de radioprotection et de sûreté nucléaire. France: Recommendations and procedures for preparedness and health surveillance of populations affected by a radiation accident. [internet, cited 2024 July 15] Available from: https://www.irsn.fr/FR/Actualites_presse/Actualites/Documents/IRSN_Shamisen-recommendation-guide_201709.pdf.
40. Clero E, et al. Lessons learned from Chernobyl and Fukushima on thyroid cancer screening and recommendations in case of a future nuclear accident. *Environ Int* 146:106230, 2021.

Chapter 8
How to educate about cancer overdiagnosis?

Prior to the development of high-resolution imaging (ultrasound and computerized tomography), most malignant neoplasms were detected after they became clinically evident. Thus, a cancer diagnosis was associated with the need for surgery or medical treatment, and the diagnosis meant significant morbidity or death. Traditionally, physicians have been taught that cancers inevitably progress in a step-wise fashion, acquiring genetic and epigenetic changes that allow for invasion and metastases to develop over a period of years. Via both clinical guidelines and the media, healthcare providers and the general public have been informed that the best prevention of cancer-related death is early detection. It is difficult to modify enthusiasm for screening after repeated broadcasting of the "early detection is the best protection" mantra. Yet, efforts are being made to educate the public about overdiagnosis, screening risks, and the variables involved in assessing risk for radiation-associated cancers.

Some experts involved in the Fukushima thyroid examination program which includes thyroid ultrasound examination (TUE) became concerned that this program was causing both overdiagnosis and early detection of indolent cancers that would not become clinically significant for a long period. These experts feared that the harms of the TUE might outweigh the benefits. Also, it became apparent that many people mistakenly believed that a TUE could determine the degree of radiation exposure and that radiation was causing thyroid cancer in Fukushima. As described in the previous chapters, believing that education is essential to helping children and preventing harm, Midorikawa, Ohtsuru, and colleagues developed educational strategies to inform participants and caregivers about the thyroid examination and thyroid cancer, including discussions of overdiagnosis and its potential harms.

Table 8-1 lists some concepts related to juvenile thyroid cancer and overdiagnosis that are poorly understood by the general public and need to be addressed via educational programs. This chapter reviews important concepts regarding thyroid cancer and discusses the methods used by Japanese endocrinology and radiation experts to inform children and adults about juvenile thyroid cancer, radiation effects, and the TUE.

Table 8-1 Juvenile thyroid cancer and overdiagnosis: What we need to understand

1. Natural history of juvenile thyroid cancer[1]

   There is now evidence that the most common type of thyroid cancer (classical papillary thyroid carcinoma) develops early in life and actively proliferates for a period of years; however, most undergo growth arrest or regression before reaching a stage of clinical significance. A small number do progress, but nearly all of these are curable or manageable after clinical manifestations occur. Deaths from juvenile thyroid cancer are extremely rare, typically occurring decades after diagnosis. These cancers are quite different from aggressive thyroid neoplasms that develop in elderly people.

2. Early diagnosis and early treatment have no proven benefits[2]

   At this time, there is no data to prove that early diagnosis and early treatment of juvenile thyroid cancer improves the survival rate or reduces the recurrence rate.

3. Medical ethics[3-5]

   Planning of research projects should involve consideration of potential risks as well as benefits, and consent forms should state the purpose of the study. Subjects should be informed when a study's purpose is to increase general knowledge that may not directly benefit participants. Participation must be purely voluntary. Subjects should have the rights to freely refuse participation and to quit participation at any time without penalty. The desire to generate new knowledge should not take precedence over the rights and interests of participants. Children have rights as human beings and should be allowed to participate in decisions regarding participation commensurate with age and maturity. When risks are found to outweigh benefits, physicians must decide whether to continue, modify or immediately stop the study. Decisions should prioritize the well-being of participants over researchers' interests. Any project that increases risk of overdiagnosis without proven health benefits should be considered a human rights issue because overdiagnosis has potential for significant harm, especially in children.

4. Harm of diagnosing juvenile thyroid cancer[6]

   The very act of diagnosing a subclinical cancer in a child or adolescent can cause serious harm. This harm cannot be avoided or mitigated by performing limited surgery or even by implementing active surveillance (AS). The diagnosis alone labels the child as a cancer patient who must carry this diagnosis into adulthood and face a prolonged period of monitoring with the risk of anxiety, depression, and stigmatization.

5. Popularity paradox[7]

   Screen-detected, subclinical thyroid cancers generally have excellent outcomes, leading patients to believe that their lives have been saved by screening. Thus, these patients have very positive views of screening and promote its value. In fact, what may be happening is that high-resolution screening is detecting mostly self-limiting or slow-growing "cancers" that will never cause clinical disease (overdiagnosis). This enthusiasm for tests that are causing harm via overdiagnosis has been called the "popularity paradox."

Section 1
Teaching about overdiagnosis in medical and allied health schools

1. Need for education of physicians and medical students

The concepts of uncertainty, probability, and overdiagnosis are often neglected in medical education. There is a need to help young doctors learn these concepts to have meaningful discussions with patients while respecting patients' values and allowing patients informed autonomy in their choices for testing and treatment.

There needs to be more discussion about what and how to teach overdiagnosis in medical education. More recently, a review article and an original article using semi-structured interview techniques on educating medical students about overdiagnosis have been published by the same group.[8, 9] The authors noted that although they recognize the need for medical education on overdiagnosis, there is no consensus on its methods. They also observed that seeking the correct diagnosis in medical education culture tends to separate from patients' values of diagnosis and to go away from addressing overdiagnosis.

The evolution of the term "overdiagnosis" from misclassification to its current meaning has coincided with changes in medical care. This includes lowering the numerical test cutoffs for diagnosis of some diseases and, in the case of cancer overdiagnosis, the use of high-resolution imaging and screening tests. Although aggressive cancers will present as or rapidly progress to clinically significant neoplasms, many incidental or screen-detected cancers will remain subclinical for a lifetime. Most of these indolent tumors are well-differentiated neoplasms with low proliferation rates; however, it is impossible to predict with 100% certainty which subclinical cancers will progress. Herein lies the need for clinicians and patients to understand the concept of probability of progression, the consequences if the neoplasm is followed without treatment, and the harms of overdiagnosis. There is a great need for medical students and practitioners to understand the concept of overdiagnosis, respect the rights of patients including older children, and develop the ability to have meaningful discussions with their patients.

Papillary thyroid carcinoma (PTC) in the young is especially vulnerable to overdiagnosis via high-resolution screening owing to its exceptionally indolent behavior and tendency to undergo growth arrest in early adulthood. Highly aggressive thyroid cancers, for example, anaplastic carcinoma, are exceptionally rare in children and typically present in older adults.[10] Whether these aggressive thyroid tumors derive via tumor dedifferentiation or evolve from a primitive ancestor is still being debated, and not a single case was reported that a small indolent PTC turned into an anaplastic carcinoma during AS.[11-14] However, even if one believes that aggressive thyroid carcinoma can evolve from a subset of differentiated thyroid carcinoma, the age differences in the onset of classical PTC versus anaplastic carcinoma, the excellent prognosis of PTC, the probability of growth arrest in PTC and evidence that PTC overdiagnosis can cause significant harm cannot be disputed. There is now evidence that overdiagnosis of juvenile thyroid cancer is occurring throughout the world.[15] True, we cannot predict on an individual patient basis which subclinical PTC will progress, but we can explain that there is, as yet, no conclusive evidence that early detection of subclinical juvenile PTC saves lives, and many harms can occur owing to unnecessary surgery, psychologic stress, and cancer-labelling with potential for lifelong stigmatization. There is a need for more medical education and for more physicians to give voice to the harm that they have witnessed.

2. Materials for the education of medical students

The Japan Consortium of Juvenile Thyroid Cancer (JCJTC) publishes online information designed to inform the general public, medical health professionals, and students about the thyroid examination and overdiagnosis. Included in this information are two videos involving medical students.

The first video shows a discussion between Toru Takano (Rinku General Medical Center) and two medical students.[16, 17] Takano reviews the situation of the Fukushima thyroid examination. He explains that most of the tumors being detected will either never progress to clinical relevance or become clinically apparent 5 or 10 years later. The prognosis of juvenile thyroid cancer is excellent, with 30-year survival >99% and lifetime survival >95%. He tells the students that only two thyroid experts in Japan publicly say that the thyroid examination is causing harm to children, yet hundreds of others remain silent or support the project.

The students are then asked what they would do if they were performing the examination. Although both students express the opinion that it would be good to stop or limit the examination, they recognize how difficult this would be given both Fukushima residents' and the TUE officials' support for the examination. They feel that they cannot do anything if their boss supports the examination and they recognize that speaking out against the exam could result in retaliation. They also state that since the examination is already underway on a large scale, it is very difficult to stop it in the middle.

The discussion gives medical students some insight into the problem of thyroid cancer overdiagnosis and points out two real problems. 1. Once a major project has been initiated, is supported by many upper-level officials, and subjects believe that they are benefiting, it is difficult to stop the project. 2. Voices in the minority are often not heeded, and sometimes there is backlash against dissenters.

The second video is a presentation by a Japanese nursing student who, as a 10-year child in Fukushima prefecture, participated in the thyroid examination.[18] When she was a high school student and later, as a nursing student, she did extensive research on the thyroid examination. In the video, she explains the lack of information given to both children and caretakers in regard to the in-school examination. Then, she discusses how she had separately and objectively informed high school students in Japan and France, respectively, about the thyroid examination including its pros and cons. After the discussion, the students are asked for their opinions about the continuation of the thyroid examination.

At the end of the video, she discusses the need for modifications in the thyroid examination. These modifications include a not-at-school venue, full disclosure of potential harms and benefits, and completely voluntary participation with no pressure to conform. Anxious individuals should be allowed to consult one-on-one with physicians rather than in a school setting. This video gives insight into the ethical issues of the examination and the Japanese culture of conformity. It also raises the question of children's rights to participate in decision-making.

Thus, the JCJTC is trying to educate medical students and the general public about the ethics of research projects and overdiagnosis. Ideally, modules dealing with these subjects should be incorporated into medical training with post-training follow-up from those in practice.

Section 2
How does one implement educational change in academic societies?

Japan is a world leader in recognition of the self-limiting/indolent behavior of papillary thyroid microcarcinoma (PMC) in adults and the advantages of non-surgical follow-up of tumors with low-risk cytological and clinical features. The safety of AS for adults with low-risk PMC has now been well-demonstrated.[19] Only a small percentage of PMCs show significant growth or develop new metastases. Delay in surgery has not been shown to worsen prognosis. Thus far, no cases of PMC followed by AS have transformed into anaplastic carcinoma or other aggressive subtypes. Gradually, AS is becoming an option for the management of low-risk PTC in adults worldwide, although the clinical criteria for low-risk tumors and enthusiasm for non-surgical follow-up vary with different countries and with different clinicians' and patients' personal beliefs, respectively.[20, 21] Concomitantly, there has been recognition of the harms of ultrasound (US) screening for thyroid cancer in asymptomatic adults. Thus, thyroid-related academic societies now acknowledge the potential for overdiagnosis and overtreatment of adult PTC and consider AS acceptable in certain circumstances.

Thyroid carcinoma in children and adolescents, however, is a different matter. It is well known that PTC in children is often associated with subclinical regional lymph node metastases and, although less commonly, distant metastases. Thus, some experts opine that US-detection of subclinical thyroid cancer is not overdiagnosis, and the executives in Japanese thyroid-related societies repeatedly emphasize the need for and safety of the thyroid examination and continue to promote it.[22-24] However, there is evidence to suggest that many of these cancers will not progress to clinical disease and that nearly all that progress can be managed successfully after progression occurs.[1] Japanese thyroid-related academic societies avoid providing opportunities to discuss overdiagnosis and criticisms of the thyroid examination in Fukushima are silenced. It has proven difficult to initiate discussions about the problems of juvenile thyroid cancer screening.

The authors propose the following:

1) Arguments from both sides of the controversy should be heard without prejudice. Those who believe that the harms of the thyroid examination are substantial should publish evidence-supported manuscripts in international journals in collaboration with overseas experts.
2) Japanese thyroid-related academic societies should welcome dispassionate discussions on both sides of the controversy and provide forums wherein both expert members and the public, including examinees and their caretakers, can discuss concerns and problems. The views of the nursing student who had been a Fukushima examinee should be heard by academics and by her fellow Fukushima residents, and debates should be initiated.[18]
3) A new academic organization that has no ties to existing academic societies or political activism should be established. Its mission will be to provide unbiased, evidence-based information that includes the views of international experts who have no conflicts of interest or political agendas. The JCJTC has played such a role to some extent. However, it currently relies on the volunteers of each member to

operate. Thus the participation of more members is necessary, as well as budgetary support.

South Korean physicians have made some progress in reducing thyroid cancer overdiagnosis through patient education and by revising US criteria for recommending fine-needle aspiration cytology (FNAC).[25-28] However, enthusiasm for US thyroid cancer screening is still strong in Korea despite efforts to discuss overdiagnosis with participants.[29] There is more work to be done worldwide. There is a need for meaningful input from academic physicians and their associated societies to minimize harm and confront one-sided messaging advocated by commercial marketing or social activists.

Section 3
How to and what to discuss with the public, residents, and patients to make them understand overdiagnosis: From the experience in Fukushima

1. People tend to overestimate the benefits of screening and medical intervention

Medical screening is defined as testing asymptomatic populations for the risk of disease and carries with it the intuitive belief that early detection of potentially life-threatening diseases, followed by early medical or surgical intervention, saves lives. The harms of screening are less well understood and acknowledged. Both clinicians and patients tend to overestimate the benefits and underestimate the harms of medical interventions including screening.[30, 31] Mass media promotion of screening sends the message that screening is the best defense against cancer. Such promotion has the financial benefits of increasing the use of US and computed tomography (CT) scanning. Promotion leads many people to believe that screening is an obligation to family and that foregoing testing is irresponsible.[32]

Fears of radiation-induced thyroid cancer contribute to the enthusiasm for thyroid cancer screening in Japan. Studies of the atomic bomb and Chornobyl accident survivors have shown that there is an increased incidence of thyroid cancer in people exposed to radiation in early childhood and infancy. Thus, the thyroid examination in Fukushima was initiated in an attempt to alleviate fears of radiation-induced cancer (see Chapter 2). Later, once thyroid cancers were detected, the optimistic belief arose that early detection with either surgical treatment or AS has benefits. Potential harms were not considered. It is very difficult to alter this mindset. Below are some possible countermeasures to educate people about overdiagnosis. Some of these were actually tried in Fukushima.

2. Use of explanatory meetings for parents and other residents with the intent to reduce anxiety

In late 2012, shortly after the initiation of the thyroid examination, Midorikawa and Ohtsuru began the implementation of face-to-face meetings with Fukushima residents in attempt to reduce anxiety.

Prior to the thyroid examination program, none of Fukushima residents had ever undergone thyroid US screening, and they were unfamiliar with the significance of US findings. Initially, explanations focused on what thyroid US can reveal and the meaning and significance of thyroid cysts and nodules. However, as described in the previous chapters, as thyroid cancer continued to be detected in the thyroid examination, the residents began to feel a new and greater fear. Therefore, it became necessary to explain more about cancer, including the natural history of thyroid cancer, its relationship to radiation exposure, and the screening effect. An attempt was made to present information in an objective fashion rather than to use wording that reflected only the presenter's values. Hino *et al.* reported that explanatory meetings regarding the effects of radiation on the thyroid gland reduced anxiety among the adults surveyed.[33]

As discussed previously, there is a general concept that early detection of cancer is beneficial, and the residents in Fukushima had not been provided with information regarding thyroid cancer and the risk-benefit ratios of screening prior to initiation of the thyroid examination. Although the surge of overdiagnosed thyroid cancer that followed US screening in Korea were discussed, it proved difficult for the residents to understand and accept that screening can have disadvantages. In response to the perceived need to provide a more detailed discussion of the benefits and harms of screening and educate the residents about radiation, the thyroid gland, and cancer, explanatory meetings were modified from 2015.

In 2018, twelve explanatory meetings on thyroid cancer were held for a total of 194 members of a consumer cooperative association. Participants were asked a few anonymous questions about the thyroid examination before and after the meeting (questionnaire response rate: 87.1%; females: ~70%; Fukushima children's caregivers: about 50%). Before the meeting, about 80% of the respondents were unaware of any possible harm as a result of thyroid cancer screening, and they believed that the benefits greatly exceeded any negative effects. Before the explanatory presentation, only 2% of the respondents did not want their children to participate in thyroid cancer screening, 72 % wanted their children to participate, and 26 % could not decide. After the meeting, these percentages changed to 33%, 36%, and 31%, respectively, because the participants became aware of the potential harms of US thyroid screening and the very low risk of radiation exposure in Fukushima. Midorikawa reported some of the results of this survey at the International Symposium in Fukushima City in 2019. These results suggest that the absence of adequate information has led to maximizing the number of TUE participants for survey subjects.

In the explanatory meetings, it was realized that certain evidence–based information is essential to understanding overdiagnosis. The general population needs to know that all cancers are not alike. Different types of cancers have distinct clinical courses, prognoses, and risk for aggressive behavior. Thyroid cancers associated with radiation generally have excellent prognoses and typically arise after a lag period of at least 4-5 years post-radiation exposure. When educating the general population about overdiagnosis, it is important that attendees at explanatory sessions understand the above information.

3. Use of classroom dialogues with children

In Fukushima, classroom dialogues were conducted in over 100 schools. On the basis of in-class conversations with school children, the following information was obtained.[34, 35] 1) Most of the children did not understand why they were supposed to undergo thyroid cancer screening; 2) many children had the misconception that the thyroid US examination (TUE) would confer personal health benefits; 3) many children had a positive impression of screening, and believed that the results could help them in the future; and 4) some children who did not actually want to receive screening participated because their parents worried about their health.

These classroom dialogues showed that about 60% of elementary school students tended to view the thyroid examination positively as something that would lead to peace of mind. Additionally, some junior high school students viewed the thyroid examination positively because they believed that the examination results could provide reassurance that cysts would not turn into cancer and as proof that Fukushima is safe. Some students, however, viewed the TUE negatively, not because they understood the disadvantages of screening but because the results might cause anxiety. The children's participation in thyroid cancer screening tended to be based on a positive impression of such examinations, a sense of social duty, and regard for their parents' anxiety. However, they were unaware of the differences in health risks posed by exposure to high versus low doses of radiation. They were also unaware of the harms of thyroid US screening.[36]

Some high school students in Fukushima were interested in radiation and its health effects and conducted various research activities during a high school science seminar. Some of them were interested in the thyroid examination and researched thyroid cancer and screening.[18]

4. Need for personal interaction with subjects

The International Agency for Research on Cancer (IARC) for Thyroid Health Monitoring after Nuclear Accidents (TM-NUC) recommends individual monitoring following certain degrees of radiation exposure.[37] Monitoring involves the selection of participants based on risk assessment rather than mass population screening. Each participant should be provided with decision aids containing adequate information on the benefits and harms of monitoring. This information should be provided by highly qualified healthcare professionals. After involvement in shared decision-making, participation should be purely voluntary. Thus, monitoring involves "education to improve health literacy" and an opt-in rather than opt-out format. Experiences of experts directly involved in the thyroid examination in Fukushima have found that personalized, face-to-face meetings with affected individuals are required in order for the residents to understand the potential harms of thyroid US including overdiagnosis.

Whether consent to participate in an activity is made via an opt-in or opt-out basis significantly impacts decision-making. Rates of consent for post-mortem organ donation are higher in countries that utilize an opt-out format as compared to an opt-in format.[38] Post-mortem organ donation cannot harm the donor and is intended to benefit the recipient; thus, an argument can be made in favor of an opt-out format. In cases of screening where there is the potential for significant harm to the examinee, the use of an opt-out format has ethical issues, and informed consent, shared decision-making, and a purely voluntary opt-in format is justified even if it results in lower rates of participation.

Moreover, the context in which the screening is offered significantly impacts decision-making. When screening is offered as a disaster response with the aim of providing support for the residents, as in the case of the thyroid screening in Fukushima, affected subjects tend to favor participation.

5. Necessity of debating harms and benefits

The World Health Organization (WHO) regional office of Europe short guide for screening programs recognizes the necessity of carefully weighing the harms and benefits of screening prior to initiation of screening projects.[39] There are potential harms associated with all screening; however, careful analysis prior to and after initiation of projects is necessary in order to ensure that harms do not outweigh the benefits, that all subjects have been adequately informed prior to participation, and that there should be neither coercion to participate nor punishment for discontinuing screening.

Also, according to Wilson and Jungner's principles of screening, "The natural history of the condition, including development from latent to declared disease, should be adequately understood."[40] Thus, participants in any screening program must be made aware of potential harms (including overdiagnosis) as well as benefits (such as early detection of certain progressive diseases). In addition, planners and organizers of screening programs are obligated to carefully analyze the harm/benefit ratios and adequately follow up and record patient outcomes. This analysis should be performed prior to and during the project to assess for the need to stop or modify the program.

The problem is that such discussions have not been held in public in Fukushima. Administrators in charge of the thyroid examination in Fukushima, therefore, need to assess whether the natural history of juvenile thyroid cancer was adequately understood prior to initiation of the thyroid examination and whether the harms of overdiagnosis, overtreatment, and psychosocial distress had been considered. After such assessment, the needs for modification of the program should be considered and implemented as deemed necessary, and reasons for changes should be honestly and openly discussed with the Japanese public. Methods should also be in place to objectively educate participants regarding harms as well as benefits. Areas of uncertainty, such as the risk of thyroid cancer progression and benefits of early treatment, should be humbly, openly, and honestly discussed. If the thyroid examination problems remain unaddressed and the project unchanged, posterity may remember the thyroid examination as a mistake that is bitterly regretted.

6. Use of social media to educate the public

The Fukushima thyroid examination, which was launched with great fanfare and with a huge budget, created various conflicts of interest. As a result, even though concerns arose that overdiagnosis was causing health damage, the government and academic societies promoting the examination were unable to acknowledge the existence of the damage. This has created an atmosphere, especially among experts, to avoid publicly discussing the problem of overdiagnosis.

When overdiagnosis of thyroid cancer occurred in South Korea, some well-meaning experts collaborated with the mass media to carry out an "anti-overdiagnosis campaign," which served as an opportunity for the public to understand overdiagnosis.[26]

On the other hand, the Japanese mass media has been reluctant to report on the problem of overdiagnosis. Some media outlets have even criticized experts who point out the harm of the examination, saying they are trying to stop the examination and cover up the health damage caused by the nuclear plant accident. Under these circumstances, it was difficult for experts to express their concerns about the Fukushima thyroid examination publicly, and as a result, the general public was denied the opportunity to understand overdiagnosis.

In an effort to overcome this situation, several Japanese thyroid specialists decided to use the anonymity of social media to inform the general public about the thyroid examination in Fukushima, and established Save Children from Overdiagnosis (SCO). At the JCJTC symposium, SCO representative Koujo Mamoru talked about the lessons learned from its activities as follows.[41] 1) It is easier to be accepted if it simply conveys the facts rather than using strong emotional or critical language. 2) Timely dissemination is important; when a topic that attracts attention in the mass media comes up, it is easier to spread the information by providing the topic in a way that matches it. 3) Different generations use different social media, and it is effective to spread information using various media. SCO started its activities in 2020, and at first, each time it disseminated information, there was a critical reaction from people who did not yet understand overdiagnosis. However, as of 2024, such criticism is scarce. It only comes from a few people with specific political backgrounds. SCO's activities are achieving certain results.

7. What should we discuss with patients?

We found no information in the literature regarding discussions of overdiagnosis with patients who have already received a cancer diagnosis and undergone therapy. Admittedly, such discussions would be tough. Such dialogues post-therapy would be expected to trigger negative reactions. Some patients might believe that their diagnoses are being trivialized or that they are being blamed for choosing to be screened, diagnosed, and treated. Others might feel that their doctors have harmed them by providing or recommending unnecessary and potentially harmful therapy. The most positive course of action at this point may be to tell patients that because their tumor was diagnosed in a subclinical stage, the prognosis is excellent. The tumor might not have progressed, but we just cannot know for sure.

Discussions of the risks of screening, the significance of subclinical neoplasia, and the probability of poor outcome are best begun before consent for screening or, in the case of incidentalomas, shared decision-making prior to biopsy or FNAC. After biopsy or FNAC, shared decision-making regarding surgical therapy versus AS for certain types of subclinical low-risk cancers would be a reasonable next step. Nonetheless, the results of such discussions have been mixed depending on participants' levels of education, health literacy, and pre-conceived faith in the benefits of screening. Many people are willing to accept the potential harms of overdiagnosis in favor of testing (popularity paradox). [7, 42]

8. Patients' and clinicians' discomfort with overdiagnosis discussion

Because cancer overdiagnosis is an epidemiological concept, it is impossible to determine, on a case-to-case basis, whether an individual has been overdiagnosed, necessitating carefully worded discussions of probability, uncertainty, and harms of overtreatment. Care must be taken not to appear to trivialize patients' fears or criticize past decisions so as not to anger or upset patients. The popularity paradox may have led patients to believe that their diagnosis would be life-saving.[7] They could feel that their doctor is denying them the right to essential care or that the health establishment is attempting to save money by trying to dissuade people from undergoing screening. Physicians are faced with the difficult task of talking about the risks and uncertainty while letting patients know that their doctor cares about them and is respecting their values, views, and autonomy.

Discussion of the overuse of imaging is problematic. Physicians may feel uncomfortable and members of the community distrustful or angry when confronted with suggestions that overuse of imaging may be harmful, even when there are pre-existing guidelines against such use.[43] Discussion and education can affect some degree of change. One can only hope that over the course of time, physicians will acquire more skill at discussing the harms of overdiagnosis and overuse of sensitive technology, and there will be incorporation of overdiagnosis and overtreatment problems into medical school curricula.

One hopes that continuing community education will allow for better informed decisions in regard to screening programs and overuse of high resolution imaging. In the case of juvenile-onset thyroid cancer, such discussions are of utmost importance because of the considerable risk for overdiagnosis and overtreatment of indolent or self-limiting neoplasms.

9. Complicated situation in Fukushima

The thyroid examination in Fukushima has raised two different issues that are of concern. The first is whether radiation exposure is the cause of increasing numbers of thyroid cancers (predominantly PTC) being detected. The second is whether the majority of the detected cancers will inevitably become clinically significant. It is important for the public to understand the following: 1) Most experts now believe that Fukushima residents' exposure to radiation was at a very low level, and the risk of radiation-induced thyroid cancer is extremely low. 2) There is now evidence that subclinical thyroid cancers occur in children who have not been exposed to radiation, and detection of juvenile thyroid cancer and overdiagnosis is increasing worldwide.

Both radiation-associated and spontaneous PTCs in the young have a low risk for morbidity and mortality, and both are susceptible to overdiagnosis. There is a need to continue to inform the residents and the general public that the detection rates of thyroid cancer in the thyroid examination are unlikely to be indicative of radiation exposure and that overdiagnosis can occur regardless of whether tumors are associated with radiation or spontaneous.

As discussed in Chapter 7, the media presentation of the TUE controversy is contributing to public confusion. It is essential that Fukushima residents and other concerned individuals have discussions with physicians and radiation experts who are trained to explain the concepts of risk, probability, uncertainty, and overdiagnosis in language that can be understood by the general public. These discussions should be aimed at engendering trust and convincing the public that these physicians and radiation experts truly care about their mental and physical well-being.

10. Summary

Efforts should be made to educate both physicians and the public about the facts and myths regarding nuclear accidents. There must be attempts of individual training to identify biased, inaccurate, and fear-mongering reports via the media and anti-nuclear activist groups. Also, there must be more opportunities for personalized patient-physician discussions, and physicians should be trained to conduct such discussions in an objective fashion while maintaining respect for patients' personal values and concerns. Heed should be given to the WHO regional office of Europe short guide for screening programs statements regarding re-evaluation of screening programs where its harms may be outweighing risks of disease.[39]

References

1. Takano T. Overdiagnosis of juvenile thyroid cancer: Time to consider self-limiting cancer. ***J Adolesc Young Adult Oncol*** 9:286-8, 2020.

2. Hay ID, *et al.* Papillary thyroid carcinoma (PTC) in children and adults: Comparison of initial presentation and long-term postoperative outcome in 4432 patients consecutively treated at the Mayo Clinic during eight decades (1936–2015). ***World J Surg*** 42:329–42, 2018.
3. General Assembly of the World Medical Association. World Medical Association Declaration of Helsinki: ethical principles for medical research involving human subjects. ***J Am Coll Dent*** 81:14-8, 2014.
4. United Nations: Convention on the Rights of the Child. [internet, cited 2024 July 15] Available from: https://www.ohchr.org/en/instruments-mechanisms/instruments/convention-rights-child.
5. Murakami M, *et al.* Harms of pediatric thyroid cancer overdiagnosis. ***JAMA Otolaryngol Head Neck Surg*** 146:84, 2020.
6. Takano T. Overdiagnosis of juvenile thyroid cancer. ***Eur Thyroid J*** 9:124-31, 2020.
7. Raffle AE, Gray JAM. Popularity paradox. In: Screening: evidence and practice. Oxford University Press, p.68, 2007.
8. Edmiston N, *et al.* Teaching to address overdiagnosis. ***BMJ Evidence-based Medicine*** doi 10.1136/bmjebm-2023-112576, 2024.
9. Colbert L, *et al.* Medical students' awareness of overdiagnosis and implications for preventing overdiagnosis. ***BMC Medical Education*** 23:256, 2024.
10. Abe I, Lam AKY. Anaplastic thyroid carcinoma: Updates on WHO classification, clinicopathological features and staging. ***Histo Histopathol*** 36:239-48, 2021.
11. Kondo T, *et al.* Pathogenetic mechanisms in thyroid follicular-cell neoplasia. ***Nat Rev Cancer*** 24:292-306, 2006.
12. Takano T. Natural history of thyroid cancer. ***Endocr J*** 64:237-44, 2017.
13. Capdevila J, *et al.* Early evolutionary divergence between papillary and anaplastic thyroid cancers. ***Ann Oncol*** 29:1454-60, 2018.
14. Dong W, *et al.* Clonal evolutionary analysis of paired anaplastic and well-differentiated thyroid carcinomas reveals shared common ancestor. ***Genes Chromosomes Cancer*** 57:645-52, 2018.
15. Vacarella S, *et al.* Global patterns and trends in incidence and mortality of thyroid cancer in children and adolescents: a population-based study. ***Lancet Diabetes Endocrinol*** 9:144-52, 2021.
16. Japan Consortium of Juvenile Thyroid Cancer. Japan: Thyroid Cancer Overdiagnosis: Round-table Discussion Part 1. [internet, cited 2024 March] Available from: https://www.youtube.com/watch?v=9igUFg3k244.
17. Japan Consortium of Juvenile Thyroid Cancer. Japan: Thyroid Cancer

Overdiagnosis: Round-table Discussion Part 2. [internet, cited 2024 July 15] Available from: https://www.youtube.com/watch?v=o1CK8n5_qr8.
18. Japan Consortium of Juvenile Thyroid Cancer. Japan: Thyroid Cancer Overdiagnosis 3-3: Opinion of an examinee. [internet, cited 2024 July 15] Available from: https://www.youtube.com/watch?v=7WsdED9LY0I.
19. Ito Y, Miyauchi A. Nonoperative management of low-risk differentiated thyroid carcinoma. *Curr Opin Oncol* 27:15-20, 2015.
20. Pollack R, Mazeh H. Active surveillance of thyroid microcarcinoma – can this approach be safely implemented worldwide? *J Surg Res* 258:145-52, 2021.
21. Pitoia F, Smulever A, Active surveillance in low risk papillary thyroid carcinoma. *World J Clin Oncol* 11:320-36, 2020.
22. Shimura H. Evaluations and current issues for Thyroid Ultrasound Examination program in Fukushima Health Management Survey. *J Jpn Thyroid Assoc* 12:133-8, 2021 (in Japanese).
23. Suzuki S. Practice of surgical treatment for pediatric thyroid cancer in Fukushima Prefecture. *J Jpn Thyroid Assoc* 12:139-48, 2021 (in Japanese).
24. Japan Thyroid Association. Japan: The opinion of the Japan Thyroid Association on the special topic "Considering thyroid cancer overdiagnosis" published in Vol. 12, No. 1 of the Journal of the Japan Thyroid Association (in Japanese). [internet, cited 2024 July 15] Available from: https://www.japanthyroid.jp/public/img/news/20210609_1201_2_opinion.pdf.
25. JoongAng Daily in Japanese. Korea: Thyroid cancer in Korean women is 14 times higher than in Japan. Why? (in Japanese) [internet, cited 2024 July 15] Available from: https://japanese.joins.com/JArticle/162430.
26. Fukushima Report. Japan: Conveying Korean's lessons to Fukushima: Overdiagnosis of thyroid cancer in Korea and the thyroid examination in Fukushima (in Japanese). [internet, cited 2024 July 15] Available from: https://synodos.jp/fukushima-report/21930/.
27. Ahn HS, Welch HG. South Korea's thyroid cancer "epidemic-turning the tide". *N Engl J Med* 373:24, 2015.
28. Kim NH, *et al.* Changes in diagnostic performance of thyroid cancer screening before and after the Korean thyroid imaging reporting and data system revision. *Korean J Fam Med* 43:225-30, 2022.
29. Lee S, *et al.* Responses to overdiagnosis in thyroid cancer screening among Korean women. *Cancer Res Treat* 48:883-91, 2016.
30. Hoffmann TC, Del Mar C. Patients' expectations of the benefits and harms of

treatments, screening, and tests: a systematic review. *JAMA Intern Med* 175:274-86, 2015.
31. Hoffmann TC, Del Mar C. Clinicians' expectations of the benefits and harms of treatments, screening, and tests: a systematic review. *JAMA Intern Med* 177:407-419, 2017.
32. Schwartz LM, *et al.* Enthusiasm for cancer screening in the United States. *JAMA* 291:71-8, 2004.
33. Hino Y, *et al.* Explanatory meetings on thyroid examination for the "Fukushima Health Management Survey" after the Great East Japan Earthquake: Reduction of anxiety and improvement of comprehension. *Tohoku J Exper Medicine* 239: 333-43, 2016.
34. Midorikawa S, *et al.* Psychosocial issues related to thyroid examination after a radiation disaster. *Asia Pac J Pub Health* 29: 63S-73S, 2017.
35. Midorikawa S, *et al.* Psychosocial impact of the thyroid examination of the Fukushima Health Management Survey. In: Thyroid cancer and nuclear accidents: Long-term aftereffects of Chernobyl and Fukushima (1st ed.). Academic Press, pp.165-73, 2017.
36. Midorikawa S, *et al.* Harm of overdiagnosis or extremely early diagnosis behind trends in pediatric thyroid cancer. *Cancer* 125:4108-9, 2019.
37. International Agency for Research on Cancer. Lyon, France: Thyroid health monitoring after nuclear accidents. IARC technical publication No.46. [internet, cited 2024 July 15] Available from: https://publications.iarc.fr/Book-And-Report-Series/Iarc-Technical-Publications/Thyroid-Health-Monitoring-After-Nuclear-Accidents-2018.
38. Johnson EJ, *et al.* Medicine. Do defaults save lives? *Science* 302: 1338-9, 2003.
39. World Health Organization regional office for Europe. Copenhagen, Denmark: Screening programmes: a short guide. Increase effectiveness, maximize benefits and minimize harm. [internet, cited 2024 July 15] Available from: https://apps.who.int/iris/bitstream/handle/10665/330829/9789289054782-eng.pdf.
40. World Health Organization. Geneva, Switzerland: Wilson JMG, Jungner G. Public Health Papers 34: Principe and practice of screening for disease. [internet, cited 2024 July 15] Available from : https://iris.who.int/bitstream/handle/10665/37650/.WHO_PHP_34.pdf?sequence=1 7.
41. Japan Consortium of Juvenile Thyroid Cancer. Japan: Thyroid Cancer Overdiagnosis 3-2: Use of social media. [internet, cited 2024 July 15] Available

from: https://www.youtube.com/watch?v=F34i_O7G98k.
42. Hersch J, *et al.* Women's views on overdiagnosis in breast cancer screening: a qualitative study. ***BMJ*** 346:f158, 2013.
43. Sharma S, *et al.* "I would not go to him": Focus groups exploring community responses to a public health campaign aimed at reducing unnecessary diagnostic imaging of low back pain. ***Health Expect*** 24:648-58, 2021.

Chapter 9
Summary of discussion points and proposals for the future

In the previous chapters, the authors have provided readers with a detailed description of the history of the thyroid examination in Fukushima, including why and how the examination was initiated. Also, the unexpected harmful effects of the examination on Fukushima residents were discussed. These include anxiety, guilt, and risk for overdiagnosis and overtreatment of self-limiting cancers (SLCs). Details of the personal experiences of two of the authors were also provided, including conflicts with the Fukushima Health Management Survey (FHMS) executive staffs.

In this final chapter, we summarize important concepts discussed in the book and convey our current ideas and plans for the future. We acknowledge that some of these ideas may change as more evidence-based data accumulate. There are some experts who disagree with us; however, it is our hope that our readers will use this book as a basis for future discussions about the potential harms of screening for thyroid cancer in children and adolescents.

There are cogent reasons to question the "early detection is the best protection" mantra when applied to self-limiting or indolent cancers such as papillary thyroid carcinoma (PTC). Although overdiagnosis cannot be predicted on an individual case basis, it cannot be denied that detection of subclinical PTC increases the overall risk for overdiagnosis. As described in the previous chapters, overdiagnosis is exceptionally harmful to children. Surgical complications do occur, especially following total thyroidectomy, and are especially devastating in children. Even diagnosis with active surveillance (AS) requires decades of follow-up and can lead to stigmatization and psychosocial problems.

We hope that those involved in thyroid cancer screening for research or clinical purposes will reflect on the material presented in this book and use it as a guide to the prevention of overdiagnosis and overtreatment of childhood thyroid tumors. We aim to protect children in all parts of the globe.

Section 1
What should we reflect on?

The thyroid examination in Fukushima has led to an increased diagnosis of thyroid cancer without cogent evidence that ultrasound (US) thyroid cancer screening is beneficial. Most experts conclude that estimated thyroid doses in Fukushima were too low to cause an increased risk of thyroid cancer in children and that Fukushima cannot be compared to Chornobyl.[1] Some continue to argue that radiation exposure is being underestimated and that the increase in childhood thyroid cancer found by the thyroid examination is related to the Fukushima nuclear power accident. The arguments on both sides must be supported by the best science and be free from biases related to pro- or anti-nuclear energy activism, personal interests, or profits.

It is our opinion, based on good science and without any political agenda, that radiation did not cause the epidemic of thyroid cancers being diagnosed in the FHMS. Not only do most experts estimate that the absorbed radiation levels were very low for the Fukushima accident, but as of 2020 very few Fukushima thyroid cancers have been found in children younger than five at the time of the accident.[1] Most cancers have been found in those who were older children or adolescents at the time of the accident. This is quite different from Chornobyl, where very many thyroid cancers were diagnosed at relatively early within 10 years in children younger than five years at the time of the accident. It is well-accepted that children younger than five are most susceptible to radiation-induced thyroid cancer. Our concerns are about the health and happiness of children. The primary focus of surveys, such as the FHMS should be on how to support the mental health and physical well-being of residents. Care must be taken to provide good communication and reduce radiophobia following a nuclear accident.[2]

During discussions of thyroid cancer screening in Fukushima, it is essential to consider two points that we consider to be indisputable. First, there is a considerable reservoir of subclinical PTC in both adults and children, and these cancers are susceptible to overdiagnosis and overtreatment. Second, radiation-associated PTC carries the same excellent prognosis as PTC in those not exposed to ionizing radiation levels on the normal environment. Potential for overdiagnosis occurs following US-diagnosis of both radiation-associated and spontaneous PTC. Thus, even in nuclear accidents such as Chornobyl, the harms of US screening of asymptomatic individuals likely outweigh the benefits.

As previously discussed, the International Agency for Research on Cancer (IARC) has concluded that population-based thyroid cancer screening following a nuclear accident has the potential to lead to overdiagnosis and is not recommended.[3] As discussed in Chapter 5, some opine that even a history of childhood radiation treatment or exposure should not be an indication for US screening owing to its potential to detect both benign nodules and indolent, differentiated thyroid cancers and because this practice can lead to unnecessary surgery and overdiagnosis.[4]

It is unfortunate that thirteen years after the Fukushima Daiichi nuclear power plant accident, thyroid cancer screening prevailed throughout Japan. There is no evidence of benefit to those who undergo screening whereas the screening is causing substantial harm. Here, to improve the present situations, we summarize some discussion and reflection points to be considered described in the previous chapters.

1. **The risk of overdiagnosis owing to the use of high-resolution US screening was not considered prior to the onset of the thyroid examination**

The increase in the detection of childhood thyroid cancer after the 1986 nuclear reactor accident at Chornobyl caused general anxiety among the residents of Fukushima following the 2011 nuclear accident. The Fukushima thyroid US examination was initiated with the goal of providing comfort and reassurance to the residents of Fukushima prefecture. Because experts estimated that the radiation exposure in Fukushima was much lower than that in Chornobyl, they did not expect to find any increase in childhood thyroid cancer.

2. **The concepts of subclinical, self-limiting childhood thyroid cancer and overdiagnosis had not been discussed with Fukushima residents**

They wonder, "If radiation is not the cause, why is the thyroid examination detecting increasing numbers of thyroid cancer?" Thus, instead of bringing comfort to the residents, the thyroid examination has increased the residents' anxiety and distrust of government officials and radiation experts.

3. **The importance of considering the damage caused by overdiagnosis even if there are effects of radiation exposure was not recognized**

Both radiation-associated and spontaneous PTC have excellent prognoses. Chornobyl should have taught us that although ionizing radiation in early childhood increases the risk of thyroid cancer, it has not been shown to increase the risk of dying of thyroid carcinoma. Demidchik et al.[5] reported only two deaths related to PTC out of 1078 thyroid cancer patients. However, one of these deaths was attributed to treatment-associated pulmonary fibrosis. There were nineteen deaths owing to other causes, including seven suicides. Of those in Chornobyl treated by surgical resection, we still must ask how many cases were overdiagnosed or overtreated. We also must ask how much diagnosis alone contributed to stress and the increase in suicides.

4. **Anger and fear have been further fueled by anti-nuclear activists who have used the increased detection of thyroid cancers to further their cause**
They support the continuation of US screening despite evidence that screening may be harmful and is without proven benefit.

5. **Support to meet the increasing demand for thyroid US examinations led to an increase in unnecessary examinations**
The government and academic societies have subsidized the purchase of US equipment and technical guidance for examiners in order to meet the demand for thyroid screening. These activities led to increased profits from performing thyroid US examinations.

6. **Without considering scientific evidence, FHMS officials have justified the continuation of the thyroid examination by emphasizing the consideration of the residents' feelings (in a Japanese word, "*yorisou*")**
They believe that the harms of overdiagnosis are being avoided because, in Japan, active surveillance (AS) for thyroid microcarcinoma is being implemented. Also, they ignore our lack of evidence about the clinical significance of subclinical regional or distant metastases. They have rejected making any major changes to the examination, such as increasing the minimal nodule diameter requiring a secondary examination or considering screening via physical examination rather than US.

7. **There has been dissemination of mixed messaging by mass media owing to divided opinion among experts**
This has led to public misunderstanding of the risks associated with radiation release in Fukushima and the potential harms of thyroid screening.

8. **Lack of medical ethics consideration regarding the thyroid examination**
Children are a vulnerable population, and there are ethical concerns with the thyroid examination that need to be addressed. Studies or surveys, such as the thyroid examination in Fukushima, should heed the guidelines set by the Declaration of Helsinki.[6]

9. **Public discussion of thyroid cancer overdiagnosis is hampered**
The presence of a sizable reservoir of subclinical cancers and the use of high-resolution imaging are the necessary prerequisites for overdiagnosis (see Chapter 1). Yet, physicians concerned about potential overdiagnosis and its harms have been forbidden to discuss this openly, nor were officials overseeing the thyroid examination in Fukushima willing to acknowledge that overdiagnosis is likely occurring.

Section 2
Measures to mitigate the harms of screening-induced overdiagnosis

In previous publications, three actions to prevent the expansion of overdiagnosis were proposed (Table 9-1).[7, 8] Countermeasures for overdiagnosis should be implemented in line with this proposal.

Table 9-1 Three actions to be taken to curb the expansion of thyroid cancer overdiagnosis in Fukushima

1) Expert opinions should be free from bias owing to conflicts of interest.
2) Residents should educate themselves to avoid fear and the popularity paradox epidemic.
3) All related people should prioritize protecting children from overdiagnosis harm over their own interests.

To summarize, although experts around the world are now recognizing the risk of overdiagnosis associated with screening, many influential people in Japan continue to claim that there is no overdiagnosis associated with the thyroid examination in Fukushima, and these views influence academia and public opinion. Their reasons for rejecting the risk of overdiagnosis have been discussed previously. Refusal to allow for discussions of overdiagnosis with the public has hindered concerned physicians from providing important risk information to the public. Also, in Japan, there is deep regard for experts who have contributed to thyroid examinations in Chornobyl and Fukushima, and their efforts are valued, leading many to believe that the thyroid examination in Fukushima should continue out of respect for the program's initiators.

When population-based US thyroid cancer screening of Fukushima children was initiated in October of 2011, the concept of overdiagnosis was little known, and virtually nothing was known about the prevalence of subclinical thyroid cancers in children and adolescents. The South Korean epidemic of subclinical thyroid carcinomas in adults that followed US screening was not published until 2014.[9] What was known in 2011 is that there was an increase in childhood thyroid carcinomas following the 1986 Chornobyl nuclear plant disaster. Thus, one cannot criticize the decision to start the thyroid examination in Fukushima.

What can be criticized is the failure to ensure that the screening program was completely voluntary, especially onsite elementary and secondary school screening. Also, remiss in the initial project was straightforward communication to participants and caregivers that the survey may not yield any benefits to individual participants and that the survey cannot determine the radiation dose to which any participant was exposed. The major advantage of the thyroid examination in Fukushima, thus far, has been obtaining new knowledge about the natural history of thyroid cancer.

There should have been monitoring to ensure that the Fukushima thyroid survey's harms do not outweigh its benefits. As discussed in Chapter 5, IARC experts do state that their recommendations are not aimed at ongoing studies and that final decisions regarding monitoring should lie with government and relevant authorities and societies.[10] However, the authors would like to emphasize again that this statement should not be used as an excuse for relevant researchers to refrain from re-evaluation of the thyroid examination.

Everyone should acknowledge and accept that mistakes are inevitable when dealing with new medical problems. In an ideal world, physicians and other scientists should be able to freely and honestly admit mistakes and design plans to curb the development of future harm without loss of reputation or respect. Admission of mistakes should be considered a sign of strength and moral courage. We believe that academic societies, FHMS leaders, and other involved experts should acknowledge the risk of overdiagnosis and actively implement changes to minimize the harms of thyroid US screening.

Authors' suggestions

1. Launch of a new task force

A new team of experts should be created. Members of this team should include experts in relevant specialties and ethics. Ideally, team members should have no conflicts of interest in thyroid cancer screening in either Fukushima or Chornobyl.

This team should be entrusted with the duty of performing an unbiased evaluation of the thyroid examination after a review of related Japanese and international publications and discussions with Fukushima residents who underwent thyroid screening. This team of experts will then recommend changes needed to minimize harm.

2. Accurate explanation to the public

The evaluation results and recommendations should then be carefully explained to the general public with the support of the government and the scientific community. If changes are recommended, it should be made clear to the public that the thyroid examination in Fukushima was initiated with good intentions; however, flaws and mistakes were discovered. Changes are being made to prevent harm, not to neglect the needs of Fukushima residents. It also should be made clear that the evaluation and recommendations were made by experts who have no political agenda, such as ties to pro- or anti-nuclear energy groups.

3. Additional scientific survey

We now know that a sizable number of young people harbor subclinical thyroid cancer, but we do not know its clinical significance. In Fukushima, there are about 80,000 children who have not received a thyroid US examination (TUE). It would be scientifically meaningful to investigate the rate of documented thyroid cancer that presented *clinically* in these children who are now adolescents and young adults. This rate should then be compared to the current rate of clinical thyroid cancer among unscreened, age-matched young people living outside the prefecture. The results of such a study will further clarify the damage caused by overdiagnosis in Fukushima, but this should not deter us from conducting it.

Personal opinions of the authors

We believe that the thyroid examination has brought unintended harm rather than comfort to Fukushima residents, and changes should be made. Below are listed our additional but personal opinions.

1. Participation in the survey must be strictly voluntary with opt-in rather than opt-out consent. The onsite school examination should be discontinued. Children and caretakers should never have been made to feel guilt or alienation for choosing not to participate, nor be made to feel that the examination was mandatory. Nor should the

school exam have been conducted in the impersonal, factory line-like fashion described in Chapter 2.

2. Residents who desire to continue being screened have the right to do so; however, there should be face-to-face consultations both before and after screening to minimize fear and anxiety. These residents deserve honest and open information regarding potential harm, including the concept of overdiagnosis, information regarding the biology of thyroid cancer, and the uncertain significance of subclinical metastases. This information should be provided by people who have been trained to present the risks and benefits in a non-judgmental and unbiased fashion.

3. There should be a standardized database documenting follow-up and management of nodules detected by screening. Such databases can provide useful information regarding outcomes and the risk of overdiagnosis. Included in the database should be participants' personal experiences during the follow-up and management period. By sharing patient information widely while protecting personal information, rather than keeping it in the hands of a limited number of doctors, patients who suffer from overdiagnosis can receive optimal support.

4. The subsidization of US machines and training programs for thyroid cancer screening should be curbed. On the other hand, there should be more education regarding the unproven benefits and potential harm of thyroid screening, and healthcare policies that address the harm of thyroid screening are required.

5. Japanese academic societies should remove the taboo on the issue of overdiagnosis of thyroid cancer in Chernobyl and Fukushima and show a willingness to encourage public discussion. By achieving a consensus among experts, we can prevent the spread of overdiagnosis and measures can be taken for the children and young people who have already suffered damage.

6. The public should be made aware that, unlike the investigation of diseases with clinical symptoms, thyroid US and fine-needle aspiration cytology (FNAC) in asymptomatic children and adolescents can cause serious harm. Strong resistance is expected because TUEs are a major source of income for medical institutions. However, this should not deter us from sounding the alarm.

7. The most challenging task will be deciding how to deal with examinees who have been diagnosed with subclinical thyroid cancer or suffered from anxiety, stigmatization, or guilt following the examination. These individuals deserve an honest apology for mistakes and to be provided with support to improve their quality of life.

Finally, the authors of this book do not aim to support a political agenda or deprive Fukushima residents of much-needed health care. Our aim is to try to answer the question, "What can we do for the children?"

References
1. UNSCEAR. Vienna, Austria: UNSCEAR 2020/2021 report volume II. [internet, cited 2024 July 15] Available from: https://www.unscear.org/unscear/publications/2020_2021_2.html.
2. Boice JD. From Chernobyl and beyond-a focus on thyroid cancer. In: Thyroid cancer and nuclear accidents: Long-term aftereffects of Chernobyl and Fukushima (1st ed.). Academic Press, pp.21-32, 2017.
3. Togawa K, et al. Long-term strategies for thyroid health monitoring after nuclear accidents: recommendations from an Expert Group convened by IARC. *Lancet Oncol* 19:1280-3, 2018.
4. Lamartina et al. Screening for differentiated thyroid cancer in selected populations. *Lancet Diabetes Endocrinol* 8:81-8, 2020.
5. Demidchik YE et al. Post-Chernobyl pediatric papillary thyroid carcinoma in Belarus: histopathological features, treatment strategy and long-term outcome, In: Thyroid cancer and nuclear accidents: Long-term aftereffects of Chernobyl and Fukushima (1st ed.). Academic Press, pp.49-58.
6. General Assembly of the World Medical Association. World Medical Association Declaration of Helsinki: ethical principles for medical research involving human subjects. *J Am Coll Dent* 81:14-8, 2014.
7. Takano T. Overdiagnosis of thyroid cancer in Fukushima. *J Society Risk Analysis, Japan* 28:67-76, 2019 (in Japanese).
8. Takano T. Overdiagnosis of juvenile thyroid cancer. *Eur Thyroid J* 9:124-31, 2020.
9. Ahn HS, et al. Korea's thyroid-cancer "epidemic"--screening and overdiagnosis. *N Engl J Med* 371:1765-7, 2014.
10. International Agency for Research on Cancer. Lyon, France: Thyroid health

monitoring after nuclear accidents. IARC technical publication No.46. [internet, cited 2024 July 15] Available from: https://publications.iarc.fr/Book-And-Report-Series/Iarc-Technical-Publications/Thyroid-Health-Monitoring-After-Nuclear-Accidents-2018.

Afterword

The lion's share of the credit for this book and for having the courage to write it belongs to my three co-authors, Drs. Midorikawa, Ohtsuru and Takano. Their combined expertise includes clinical endocrinology, thyroid oncology and radiation biology. My experience is mainly in the field of diagnostic cytopathology. Through the years, I have developed a strong interest in preventing the harms of too much medicine. This interest was acquired after looking back at my own mistakes and my misguided enthusiasm for making diagnoses regardless of whether those diagnoses would benefit patients. Eventually, I realized that some conditions are best left undiscovered. The harms of unrestrained organ interrogation by ultrasound (US) or computerized tomography outweigh benefits. Thus, I support my co-authors' endeavors to provide information about the Fukushima Health Management Survey (FHMS) thyroid examination to physicians and other professionals outside of Japan. It has been an honor to be asked to help write this book. A few personal closing thoughts are given in the following paragraphs. Some of these thoughts reemphasize concepts discussed in previous chapters.

As we age, all physicians will witness the transformation of once sacrosanct medical practices into mistakes that are ultimately determined to be without benefit or to cause more harm than good. Historical examples include the use of the Halsted radical mastectomy for breast cancer and milk and antacid therapy for peptic ulcer disease. My more than 30-year sojourn in cytopathology has led me away from the naïve belief that finding cellular atypia or cancer via fine needle aspiration of subclinical thyroid lesions is beneficent. My initial enthusiasm has given way to remorse about misclassification and overdiagnosis of lesions best left unsampled and fear that we are continuing to perform too much unnecessary surgery. Use of high-resolution ultrasonography has steadily increased in the United States, and, concomitantly, diagnosis of and surgery for differentiated thyroid cancers, follicular neoplasms and "atypia of undetermined significance" has increased. Although the use of molecular testing (MT) is currently being touted as a means to decrease thyroid surgery in adults, it should be recognized that MT is costly and will not reduce the need for long-term follow-up or the anxiety and expense associated with this follow-up. One might make the same comments about some of our new US bells and whistles such as elastography.

It is our hope that this book will not only effect more productive conversations about thyroid cancer screening after a nuclear accident but will motivate practicing clinicians, pathologists and radiologists throughout the world to consider the potential harms incurred by US detection and overly aggressive treatment of subclinical thyroid nodules in children and adolescents. It should again be emphasized that the harms of overdiagnosis and overtreatment are much greater in children and adolescents than in adults, and also they are harmful enough in adults. It is heartening that some physicians in the United States are beginning to acknowledge that there is a problem concerning how to treat childhood thyroid neoplasms without harms outweighing benefits.[1]

Albeit there are dissenters, based on most expert assessments very few, if any, Fukushima children were exposed to radiation levels high enough to pose a major risk for thyroid cancer. However, even if a few of the more than 300 US-detected papillary thyroid carcinomas (PTCs) are radiation-related, one would not expect those children to fare any worse than those with spontaneous PTC. Several experts now question whether history of childhood radiation exposure justifies US screening for thyroid cancer.[2,3] The detrimental effects of screening even the so-called high-risk groups may well outweigh the benefits. It has not been shown that thyroid cancer survival or quality of life is improved by US screening of those who underwent childhood radiation, and US often detects benign nodules that undergo surgical excision. One worries that history of radiation exposure alone might induce some surgeons and endocrinologists to recommend excision of any detected thyroid nodule, thus contributing to our increase in unnecessary thyroid surgery.

True, metastases are very commonly detected in children with PTC; however, regardless of the presence or absence of metastases, the overall long-term prognosis for both radiation-related and spontaneous childhood PTC is excellent. We do not yet understand the significance of subclinical metastases. Thus, one must consider that the presence of US or surgically diagnosed metastases does not necessarily eliminate the possibility of overdiagnosis and overtreatment. It must also be acknowledged that total thyroidectomy and radioactive iodine therapy pose significant complication risks for children.[1,4] The concept that metastases may, in some cases, be harmless is a radical concept that is very difficult for both physicians and patients to accept. It goes against traditional cancer dogma. Should not we now revisit Cronan's 2008 question, "Is it time to turn off the ultrasound machines"[5] and refrain from US interrogation of healthy children's subclinical thyroid nodules regardless of history of- or possibility of radiation exposure?

There is a need for conversations, and we should strive to develop mutual trust between patients and their doctors. The public should know that there is no certainty in medicine, only estimated risks and probabilities. Not every patient will respond favorably to conversations about risks of screening and overdiagnosis, but that does not mean one should not try to have such conversations and let patients know that their physicians care about their well-being and happiness. We, as physicians, must learn how to talk with patients about these risks and probabilities while continuing to show respect for patients' views and autonomy. This is not easy because one must adjust conversations to differences in patients' cultures, education, numeracy, cognitive biases and, too often, prior acquisition of misinformation. Sometimes, physicians must deal with pressure to follow guidelines that are not always be in the best interest of individual patients.

Patients must be reassured that their informed personal decisions regarding screening and treatment are sacrosanct and that their physician will not judge them favorably or unfavorably based on their choices. It is also critical that the art of patient-doctor conversations about risks and probability be included in early medical student education. Perhaps this could be accomplished via simulated patient interviews or problem-based learning activities. Patients' autonomy should include freedom to decline surgery without being told by physician, family or friends "don't be stupid" or to "get the thing cut out". Pressure to have surgery after detection of an asymptomatic malignant, suspicious or atypical thyroid nodule has been reported by Davies *et al*.[6]

In Chapter 7, Midorikawa relates the story of a young man who opted for thyroidectomy so as not to make his mother sad. Young people should not feel compelled to undergo surgery because of filial compassion rather than presence of clinical indications. Perhaps, both the patient and his mother would have been comforted had adequate informed consent been given and overdiagnosis risk discussed prior to screening. Perhaps, then, if they so desired, they would have felt free to decline screening without experiencing guilt, alienation, or loneliness.

Many non-thyroid cancer screening programs are controversial as to risk-benefit ratios, especially in certain age groups. Mammography, prostate specific antigen testing, and low-dose computerized lung cancer screening are examples. Physicians, other healthcare professionals and commercial enterprises tend to emphasis the benefits of screening but fail to discuss risks such as false positives, overdiagnosis, and treatment-associated harms. Choosing not to undergo screening has its own problems. There can be psychosocial harms associated with refusal of testing. Schwartz *et al.* found that some considered undergoing cancer screening an obligation.[7] These findings imply that people can be seen as not being attentive to their family's happiness if they do not undergo screening. My co-authors have reported similar feelings of obligation in Fukushima parents and their children. Better and well-balanced discussions with patients, along with inclusion of family members when indicated, is required. Many will still choose screening as is their right to so do; however, those who decline screening should not be made to feel that they are inconsiderate, foolish people who do not love their families.

Another potential adverse screening effect is quality-metrics screening of doctors. Physicians should not be punished or censured because patient cancer screening participation rates do not meet benchmarks when these physicians have documented shared discussions about screening with their patients, and patients subsequentially decline screening. Such documented discussions should be considered good patient care and should not only protect physicians but also protect patients from unjustly being labelled "non-compliant".

Two of this book's authors, Drs. Midorikawa and Ohtsuru, have participated directly in the FHMS thyroid ultrasound examination (TUE) and personally witnessed the adverse effects of this examination on the children of Fukushima and their parents. They also found that children or caretakers who declined screening experienced guilt or alienation. Dr. Takano has long supported the idea that US screening of children for thyroid carcinoma is harmful and has published the argument that, while a subset of childhood PTC progress to clinical significance, childhood PTC do not directly progress into the very aggressive, lethal types of thyroid cancer found in older adults. It takes moral courage to wage academic opposition to the *zeitgeist* opinion that "early detection is the best protection" and to call for admission that honest mistakes were made.

For political reasons, as this book explains, such arguments can lead to accusations of trying to cover up the harms of radiation-induced carcinogenesis or to back-lash from those in charge. It is difficult for physicians and other scientists to openly admit mistakes and try to prevent further harm from these mistakes. Admission of mistakes and initiation of changes designed to minimize harm should be considered a respect-worthy strength. In the real world, unfortunately, fear of loss of reputation and respect, loss of monetary benefits, and fear of litigation (in countries such as the United States) are obstacles to the implementation of changes to diagnosis and treatment standards.

The authors of this book argue that the FHMS thyroid cancer screening examination has caused unpredicted and unintentional harms that now should be addressed. The project protocol should be modified, and open and honest discussions with the public are needed. None of the authors seek to cover-up dangers from radiation nor have any political agendas. The purpose of this book is not to argue in support of- or protest against the use nuclear energy. We argue that surveys such as the FHMS TUE must be continuously monitored for harms, these harms should be acknowledged, and suitable survey modifications should be made. If inaccurate or biased information is used to support a cause, no matter how worthy that cause may be, this information can harm members of a society whom one is trying to protect.

As Boice has so compellingly put it, "No one cares how much you know unless they know how much you care."[8] After working with my co-authors and having read many of their publications, it has become clear to me that they truly care about the health and happiness of Fukushima children, and I hope that, after reading this book, others will agree with me.

References
1. Shaha AR, Tuttle RM. Pediatric thyroid cancer: A surgical challenge. ***Eur J Surg Oncol*** 45:2001-2, 2019.
2. Tonorezos ES, *et al.* Screening for thyroid cancer in survivors of childhood and young adult cancer treated with neck radiation. ***Cancer Surviv*** 11:302-8, 2017.
3. Lamartina L, *et al.* Screening for differentiated thyroid cancer in selected populations. ***Lancet Diabetes Endocrinol*** 8:81-8, 2020.
4. Fridman M, *et al.* Factors affecting the approaches and complications of surgery in childhood papillary thyroid carcinoma. ***Eur J Surg Oncol*** 45:2078-85, 2019.
5. Cronan JJ. Thyroid nodules: Is it time to turn off the ultrasound machines? ***Radiol*** 247:602-4, 2008.
6. Davis L, *et al.* Experience of US patients who self-identify as having an overdiagnosed thyroid cancer: a qualitative analysis. ***JAMA Otolaryngol Head Neck Surg*** 143:663-9, 2017.
7. Schwartz LM, *et al.* Enthusiasm for cancer screening in the United States. ***JAMA*** 291:71-8, 2004.
8. Boice JD. From Chernobyl and beyond-a focus on thyroid cancer. In: Thyroid cancer and nuclear accidents: Long-term aftereffects of Chernobyl and Fukushima (1st ed.). Academic Press, pp.21-32, 2017.

Vicki J Schnadig
University of Texas Medical Branch at Galveston,
U.S.A.

Overdiagnosis of thyroid cancer in Fukushima

2024 年 10 月 11 日　初版 1 刷発行
著　者　Sanae Midorikawa, Toru Takano, Akira Ohtsuru,
　　　　Vicki J Schnadig
発行者　岡林信一
発行所　あけび書房株式会社
　　　　　　　〒 167-0054　東京都杉並区松庵 3-39-13-103
　　　　　　　☎ 03.-5888- 4142　FAX 03-5888-4448
　　　　　　　info@akebishobo.com　https://akebishobo.com

印刷・製版／モリモト印刷
ISBN978-4-87154-273-9　C3047